SURGICAL AND MEDICAL TREATMENT IN ART

Alan EH Emery and
Marcia LH Emery

Foreword by
Sir John Hanson

Dedicated to the memory of

Robert Platt,
Baron Platt of Grindleford
(1900–1978)

A renowned physician and lover of the arts

SURGICAL AND MEDICAL TREATMENT IN ART

Alan EH Emery and
Marcia LH Emery

Foreword by

Sir John Hanson

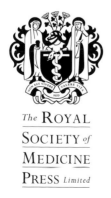

The ROYAL
SOCIETY *of*
MEDICINE
PRESS *Limited*

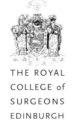

THE ROYAL
COLLEGE of
SURGEONS
EDINBURGH

Founded 1505
From here health

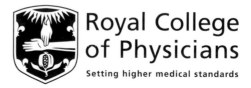

Royal College
of Physicians
Setting higher medical standards

Published by the Royal Society of Medicine Press Ltd
1 Wimpole Street, London W1G 0AE, UK
Tel: +44 (0)20 7290 2921
Fax: +44 (0)20 7290 2929
Email: publishing@rsm.ac.uk
Website: www.rsmpress.co.uk

British Library Cataloguing in Publication Data
A catalogue record for this book is available from the British Library

ISBN 1-85315-695-7

Distribution in Europe and Rest of World:

Marston Book Services Ltd
PO Box 269
Abingdon
Oxon OX14 4YN, UK
Tel: +44 (0)1235 465500
Fax: +44 (0)1235 465555
Email: direct.order@marston.co.uk

Distribution in the USA and Canada:

Royal Society of Medicine Press Ltd
c/o Jamco Distribution Inc
1401 Lakeway Drive
Lewisville, TX 75057, USA
Tel: +1 800 538 1287
Fax: +1 972 353 1303
Email: jamco@majors.com

Distribution in Australia and New Zealand:

Elsevier Australia
30-52 Smidmore Street
Marrikville NSW 2204, Australia
Tel: +61 2 9517 8999
Fax: +61 2 9517 2249
Email: service@elsevier.com.au

Typeset by Phoenix Photosetting, Chatham, Kent
Printed in the Netherlands by Alfabase, Alphen aan den Rijn

CONTENTS

FOREWORD

In this second volume by Alan and Marcia Emery, published three years after their fascinating and original, *Medicine and Art*, the authors resume their exploration of the tripartite relationship that links healers, patients and the seemingly different world of artists. It is a companion volume, but the story moves on as the focus sharpens, revealing further examination of the evolution of treatments, especially in surgery, from ancient to modern times. Intriguingly, the worlds through which the characters move turn out to be not separate after all. Physicians and surgeons are artists and artists, patients. All is not quite what it seems. But it is the human condition and it is the artist's condition to comment – as well as record.

The book is elegantly published once again by The Royal Society of Medicine Press and appears additionally under the aegis of both The Royal College of Physicians and The Royal College of Surgeons of Edinburgh. It provides sixty-six plates of great diversity to illustrate the story, which is told in the same number of admirably concise essays. There is a useful list of a hundred and fifty-four further works of art not included in the final list selected for this volume.

The authors are at pains to avoid didacticism. They do not force theories or conclusions - the style is one of restraint. Their preference is to invite and expect the reader to observe and ponder, perhaps on the breathtaking acceleration in the development of therapies in the twentieth century, on the significance of antisepsis, antibiotics and modern anaesthetics, or on the evidently mixed responses of artists to treatments. Eakins' *The Gross Clinic* and Ensor's *The Bad Doctors* may sound negative notes. Have Ken Currie's oncologists something to explain?

The Fellows of Green College take pride in Alan and Marcia Emery's *Surgical and Medical Treatment in Art*. They again provoke our questions and stimulate our thinking. They always nudge us to read on.

Sir John Hanson KCMG CBE MA
Warden, Green College, Oxford, 2005

ACKNOWLEDGEMENTS

It is a very great pleasure to acknowledge those various individuals and organizations who have kindly granted us permission to reproduce the works of art in this book, and those who have supplied images. There are many other individuals who gave us much useful help and advice and whom we should like to thank personally. They include Mr Clive Coward, Senior Picture Researcher, Historical Collection, The Wellcome Trust Medical Photographic Library; Ms Tina Craig, Deputy Head of Library and Information Services, Royal College of Surgeons of England; Ms Christine Campbell, The British Library, Permissions Department; Miss Cristina Robins, Picture Library Assistant, Royal Collection Enterprises Ltd; Dr Thorsten Opper, Curator, Department of Greek and Roman Antiquities, British Museum; Ms Joanna Bowring, Head of Libraries and Information, British Museum; Ms Jenny Crispin, Hunterian Museum; Mr John Melville, a freelance photographer; Mr Euan Mackay; and Dr Geoffrey Farrer-Brown, Chairman of the charity, *A Picture of Health*. We are also especially grateful for the help of Mr Bill Hopkins and his staff at the Department of Medical Illustration of the University of Edinburgh and Ms Clare Marks, Publications Department, Royal College of Physicians.

Special thanks are due to Dr Peter Watkins, Editor of *Clinical Medicine (Journal of the Royal College of Physicians)* and Ms Diana Beaven, Publications Manager, Royal College of Physicians of London, who first encouraged us to pursue the project of relating works of art to developments in the diagnosis, management and treatment of disease.

Most importantly, we owe a particular debt of gratitude to Mr Peter Richardson, Managing Director of the Royal Society of Medicine Press, whose enthusiastic support and encouragement has been so important, and to his colleagues at RSM Press, Ms Alison Campbell and Ms Hannah Wessely, for their professional and untiring help and advice.

Finally, we are most grateful to the Warden, Sir John Hanson, and Fellows of Green College, Oxford for providing facilities for researching and writing the book.

Oxford, 2005

INTRODUCTION

'If you would judge, understand'

Seneca, *The Dialogues*[1]

'Seeing comes before words'

John Berger, *Ways of Seeing*[2]

Much has been written on subjects of medical and surgical interest depicted in works of art. Perhaps the most notable and detailed early study was that by Paul Richer in Paris in 1887[3] and the later work written by Charcot and Richer.[4] Charcot himself was not only a renowned neurologist but also an accomplished artist who often drew his patients. Particularly interesting from the present point of view is a large section in their monograph devoted to various treatments, medical and surgical, known at the time. Since then, a number of authoritative texts on the subject have been published, and some more recent ones are listed in the references.[5–15]

A number of physicians and surgeons have themselves been artists and therefore their work is particularly of interest. They include not only Jean Martin Charcot, but also Georges-Alexandre Chicotot in France and Sir Charles Bell, Sir Francis Haden, Henry Tonks, John Wells and Sir Roy Calne in Britain. The latter is noteworthy because of his numerous paintings of his patients with a variety of surgical conditions. We include works by Chicotot and Calne in this volume.

Our aim has been to arrange paintings concerned with surgical and medical treatments roughly in the chronological order of the events depicted rather than according to the date a particular work was created. Furthermore, we have attempted to select those works that best illustrate an innovation. Towards the end of the book we have selected the work of some present-day artists, who address some of the problems and dilemmas facing the profession in its pursuit of effective treatments.

Of course, in a book limited in size we have been able to include only a fraction of all the works on the subject and, as in our previous book,[16] our selection has therefore been somewhat eclectic and much influenced by our own personal preferences. We list other examples of various surgical, dental and medical treatments in art in a Table at the end.

Several noted neuroscientists are currently exploring the brain's activity in interpreting visual images.[17,18] Various techniques, including functional magnetic resonance imaging, have revealed how different parts of the brain are involved in identifying and interpreting visual images. As Zeki[18] has so elegantly concluded:

'Knowledge of [the brain's] operations and of its products, including the works of art which have enriched our cultures and which we so admire, merely enhances the sense of wonder and beauty, because we then begin to admire not only the product but also the organ that is able to produce it'.

References

1. Seneca LA. *Dialogues and Letters*. London: Penguin Books, 1997.
2. Berger J. *Ways of Seeing*. London: BBC and Penguin Books, 1972.
3. Richer P. *L'Art et La Médecine*. Paris: Gaultier Magnier, 1887.
4. Charcot J-M, Richer P. *Les Deformes et les Malades dans l'Art*. Paris: Lecrosnier et Babé, 1889.

5.   Wilenski RH. *Dutch Paintings*. London: Faber & Faber, 1929.
6.   van Dongen JA. *De Zieke Mens in de Beeldende Kunst*. Amsterdam: De Bussy, 1968.
7.   Lyons AS, Petrucelli RJ. *Medicine: An Illustrated History*. New York: Abrams, 1987.
8.   Siraisi NG. *Medieval and Early Renaissance Medicine*. Chicago: University of Chicago Press, 1990.
9.   Carmichael AG, Ratzan RM. *Medicine in Literature and Art*. Cologne: Könemann, 1991.
10. Nuland SB. *Medicine: The Art of Healing*. New York: Macmillan, 1992.
11. Sournia J-C. *The Illustrated History of Medicine*. London: Harold Starke, 1992.
12. Downie RS (ed). *The Healing Arts: An Oxford Illustrated Anthology*. Oxford: Oxford University Press, 1994.
13. Haslam F. *From Hogarth to Rowlandson: Medicine in Art in Eighteenth Century Britain*. Liverpool: Liverpool University Press, 1996.
14. Porter R (ed). *Medicine: A History of Healing*. London: O'Mara Books, 1997.
15. Jones PM. *Medieval Medicine in Illuminated Manuscripts*. London: British Library, 1998.
16. Emery AEH, Emery, MLH. *Medicine and Art*. London: Royal Society of Medicine Press, 2003.
17. Matthews PM, McQuain J. *The Bard on the Brain*. New York: Dana Press, 2003.
18. Zeki S. *Inner Vision: An Exploration of Art and the Brain*. Oxford: Oxford University Press, 2003.

The Plates

1

Pectoral with a Heart Scarab in a Barque (Nineteenth Dynasty, c 1275 BC, Egypt)

anonymous

The ancient Egyptian civilization grew up around the Nile valley. The first truly historical period begins with the invention of writing around 3000 BC and from then until 300 BC is the Dynastic Period, a term derived from the 31 dynasties of the successive kings of Egypt. To explain and understand the origin of the universe and various other phenomena, including illness, the ancient Egyptians developed a complex mythology involving various deities. Although details varied from period to period and from place to place, certain principal characters remained generally constant throughout. The principal gods included, for example, Re (or Ra), the sun-god creator, Osiris, the king of the underworld and the dead, and Isis, the wife of Osiris.

Three other deities are relevant to this essay: Horus, the symbol of divine kingship and son of Osiris, depicted as a falcon; Seth, the god of disorder, storms and violence, represented by several different animal forms; and Thoth, the god of wisdom and learning, depicted as an ibis or baboon.

According to legend, Seth murdered his brother Osiris. To avenge this deed, Horus fought with Seth and in doing so lost an eye, which was then restored by Thoth. In this way, the eye of Horus became a symbol of completeness and perfection, known as the *wedjat*. It is depicted as a stylized human eye with cosmetic colouring and two lines drawn from the lower lid. In jewellery, the wedjat was often associated with a scarab or dung beetle, as here, and represented the sun. The left eye of Horus was a symbol of the moon and the right eye another symbol of the sun.

The wedjat became a popular protective amulet and ensured good health. The image later passed from the Egyptians to the Greeks and Arabs, and there is evidence that it may well have persisted even to the present day as a symbol or sign (R$_X$) for a medical recipe or prescription.

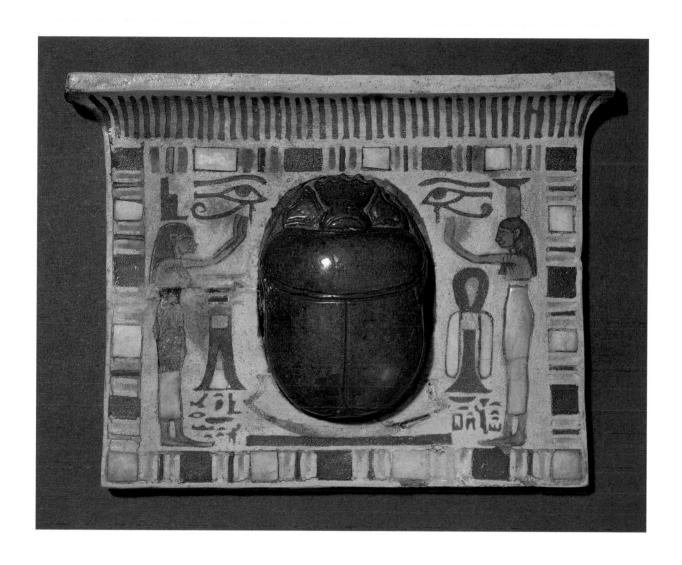

Pectoral with a Heart Scarab in a Barque (Nineteenth Dynasty, c 1275 BC, Egypt), anonymous. Polychrome glazed composition plaque. Height 9.7 cm. *London, British Museum. EA7865.*

2

Instruments in Ancient Egypt (Roman period, c AD 150–200)

temple relief, Kom Ombo, anonymous

The upper illustration is a copy commercially available to tourists in Egypt of a relief on the wall of the temple of Kom Ombo. It is a fairly faithful copy of published black-and-white photographs of the relief that dates from the time of the Roman period in Egypt (30 BC – AD 323). It depicts instruments used at the time, several of which are clearly surgical. For example, two at the bottom right-hand corner are Roman scalpels; others are clearly forceps and various types of cutting implements, including a saw with a serrated edge. It seems, however, that in Ancient Egypt only the simplest operations were performed, including circumcision, paracentesis for ascites, incision of abscesses and cysts, and occasionally skull trephination. Most surgical expertise was used in dealing with trauma. For example, wounds might be sutured and then bound with oil and honey, the latter now being known to have antibacterial properties. There is evidence that fractures were splinted and dislocations reduced by manipulation. This is shown in the lower figure, based on a painting on the wall of a tomb at Thebes around 1200 BC. Another relief shows a woman delivering a baby in a semi-sitting position, a common posture for childbearing for thousands of years and still employed in parts of Africa today.

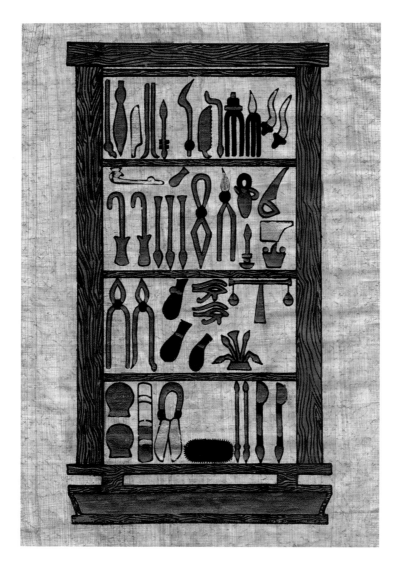

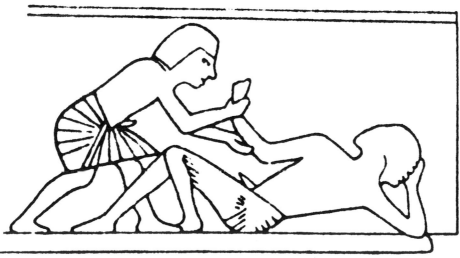

Upper figure: **Instruments in Ancient Egypt** (Roman period, c AD 150–200), anonymous. From carved temple relief at Kom Ombo. Oil on papyrus, 34 cm × 26 cm. *Author's collection.*

Lower figure: **Reduction of Dislocated Shoulder** (1200 BC), anonymous. From a wall painting, Tomb of Ipuy, Thebes.

Reproduced with permission and copyright © of The British Editorial Society of Bone and Joint Surgery.

3

Manipulation of a Joint (c 1800)

by Zhou Pei Qun

Chinese medicine has a very long history dating back well over 2000 years, with a philosophical and supernatural approach to the causes of disease. The concept of two opposing forces, *Yang* and *Yin*, dominated concepts of health and disease. Important elements in treatment included a great variety of decoctions and infusions, as well as pills and powders. Some of these were based on herbs but many on a variety of animal tissues. Many prescriptions, or *fang*, were based on thousands of combinations of these compounds, many of which are still in use in traditional Chinese medicine today.

Several physical approaches to treatment also owe their origins to Chinese medicine. These include acupuncture and moxibustion, which is analogous in some ways to cupping in the West and consisted of burning small pellets of dried wormwood at specific points on the skin. The Chinese also excelled in manipulation, which was not exclusively Chinese, having been practised in several other cultures from the earliest times. But the Chinese certainly perfected the technique, which nowadays is also related to chiropractic and osteopathy.

An important legacy of traditional Chinese medicine is reflected in today's emphasis on an holistic approach to the patient. Furthermore, it is now associated with many aspects of so-called complementary or alternative medicine. But, disappointingly, few such therapies have so far been subjected to critical analysis.

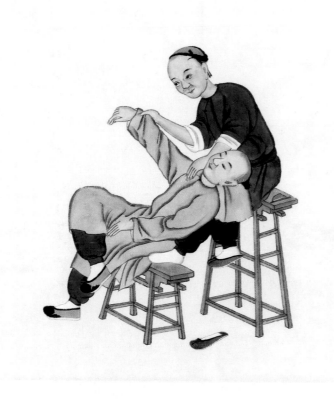

此中國剃頭棚放睡之圖也每日將頭剃完
筋骨疼痛者剃頭者坐于高橙之上其人躺
在剃頭膝上令其捶拿其快活無比

周培春畫

Manipulation of a Joint (c 1800) by Zhou Pei Qun (fl 1800). Watercolour on rice paper, 26 cm × 34.5 cm. *London, Wellcome Library.*

4

The Warrior Guan Yu Plays *Go* While the Surgeon Hua T'o Operates on His Arm (1853)

by Utagawa Kuniyoshi

The Chinese surgeon Hua T'o of the 2nd century AD, a contemporary of Galen, was much revered by his countrymen. He was famed for his skills in acupuncture and moxibustion. He was also believed to have been able to foretell the sex of an unborn child. Here, the artist has depicted an imaginary scene of the surgeon operating on the famous soldier of the period, General Guan Yu. Apparently it was expected that one should bear pain without emotion. So the general is portrayed continuing to play the board game, *Go*, while the surgeon deftly attempts to remove a poisoned arrow from his arm, which has a tourniquet around it. Nevertheless, some kind of anaesthesia was often used, including wine and drugs such as henbane (hyoscyamine) or even opium. But apart from the surgical treatment of wounds, early Chinese surgeons were opposed to any invasion of the human body and surgical interventions were not encouraged. When Hua T'o offered trephination of the skull to Prince Tsao Tsao, who was suffering from severe headaches, it was suspected the surgeon wished to murder him.

Utagawa Kuniyoshi (1797/8–1861) was in fact Japanese and one of the last great masters of woodblock print. He became particularly famous for his series *Hundred and Eight Chinese Heroes*. He was also famous for his drawings of cats, his studio being full of them. He died in Edo, now Tokyo, in 1861, just a few years after the great earthquake that had devastated the city.

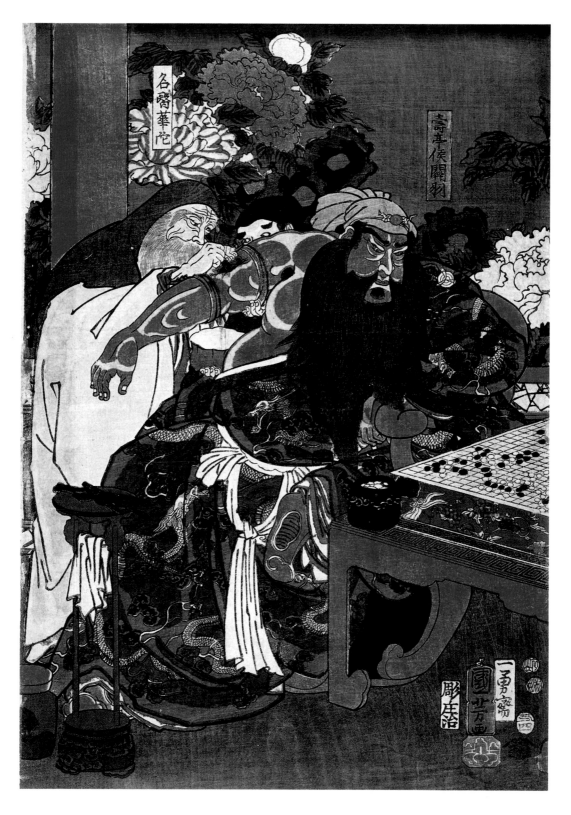

The Warrior Guan Yu Plays Go While the Surgeon Hua T'o Operates on His Arm (1853) by Utagawa Kuniyoshi (1797/8–1861). Coloured woodcut, 35.6 cm × 23.2 cm. *London, Wellcome Library.*

5

Tombstone of the Athenian Physician Jason (2nd century BC)

anonymous

This relief was found in Attica in the 18th century and eventually sold to the British Museum. According to the Sculpture Catalogue, Jason was a 2nd century Greek physician. Here he appears to be examining the swollen abdomen of a young boy who was perhaps suffering from ascites.

The first individual in the history of medicine to be credited with a rational approach to disease, rather than one based on mythological and philosophical ideas, was Hippocrates (c 460–370 BC), a Greek physician born on the island of Kos. He is credited with having written over 70 works on medical practice. Although there is some doubt about the precise authorship of these works, there is no doubt that he is the real father of modern medicine. He is remembered best for the Hippocratic Oath, of which there are numerous English translations and renderings. Important points that it contains, however, are that the physician should help the sick according to his ability, never administer a poison or give a woman any means to procure an abortion, not cut even for the stone but leave this to practitioners of the art, never physically harm or sexually abuse his patients, and whatever he sees or hears he will never divulge. Many aphorisms attributed to him contain much common sense: 'Life is short but the Art is long'.

The relationship between the physician and his young patient in this carved stone relief seems to indicate the faith and trust of the patient in his doctor.

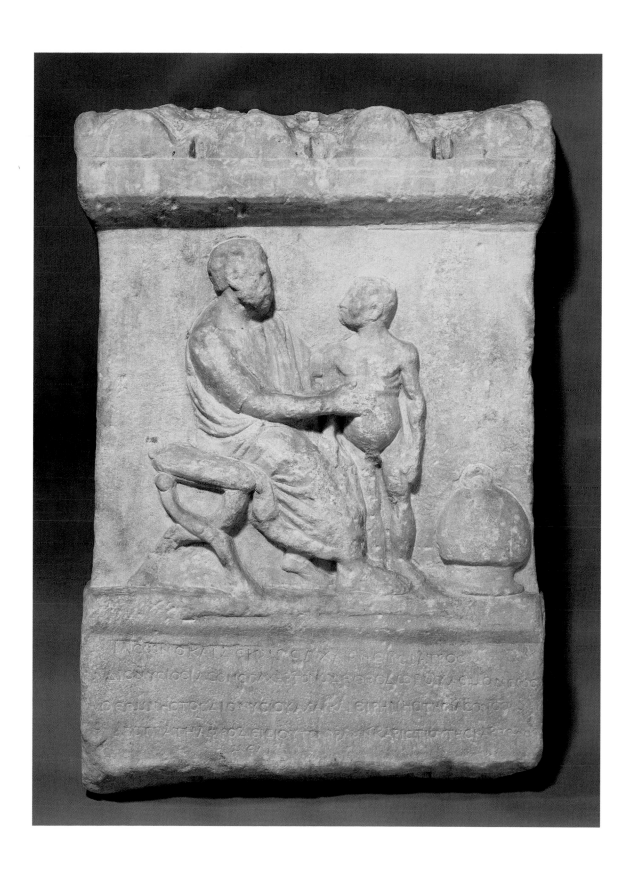

Tombstone of the Athenian Physician Jason (2nd century BC), anonymous. Greek sepulchral bas-relief, Pentelic marble, 78.7 cm × 57.2 cm. *London, British Museum. 629.*
© Copyright of the Trustees of the British Museum.

6

Cautery (c 1100)

English mediaeval illuminated manuscript

'Cautery' was a term used in two different regards. Firstly, as illustrated in this English manuscript from around AD 1100, it was a form of treatment for a variety of medical conditions and involved applying a hot iron to various parts of the body. Here, there is a brazier in which various types of cautery instruments are being heated. The physician on the left offers a beaker to the patient – perhaps a painkilling drink. Albucasis (AD 936–1013), the renowned Arabic doctor, used the technique extensively for treating a variety of internal diseases, including epilepsy, stroke and mental illness. He also describes its use for cauterizing abscesses, skin tumours and haemorrhoids.

The term was also used for applying a hot iron or scalding oil ('potential cautery') to a wound, supposedly to destroy poisons or prevent putrefaction and staunch blood flow. In this way, cautery was used for hundreds of years before eventually being condemned by Ambroise Paré in 1537. Subsequently, ligatures began to be used to stem bleeding, but this only became practical with the introduction of screw tourniquets in the 18th century by the French surgeon Jean-Louis Petit, who, incidentally, was the first to perform a successful operation for mastoiditis. But it was a very long time before electric cautery was introduced by John Caulk in the 1920s.

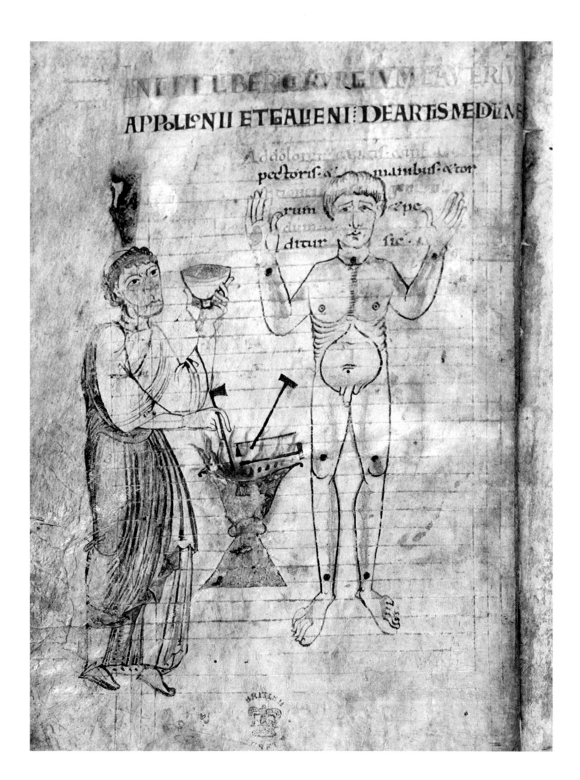

Cautery (c 1100). English mediaeval illuminated manuscript. Pen and ink and colour. *London, The British Library. Sloane, MS 2839, f1v.* By permission of The British Library.

7

Mandrake (Mandragora Root) (c 1175)

Mosan mediaeval illuminated manuscript

Opium and alcohol have long been used to deaden pain. Discorides (or Dioscurides), a Greek physician who served as a doctor in the Roman army in the first century AD, described some 600 plants and their medical uses in which he advocated the mandragora root (commonly named mandrake) steeped in wine to deaden pain, including in surgical operations. Its use continued in various ways even until the early 19th century. According to *Culpepper's Herbal* from the 17th century, it could also be used as an emetic and purgative. Botanically, it belongs to the family of Solanaceae, which includes, among other species, henbane or hyoscyamine, sometimes referred to as the 'poor man's opium'. According to legend, the mandrake root had a human shape, in two varieties, one masculine and one feminine. It shrieked terribly when dug up, which would be fatal to any man who attempted to uproot it. For this reason, a dog was hitched to the plant for the purpose of digging it up and this was a common feature of early English and German folklore. Nowadays, the plant grows in the Near East and is known to be poisonous.

The active ingredients of a number of plants used previously for various purposes were extracted in the early 19th century, leading to the isolation of several alkaloids, including morphine, codeine and cocaine. This set the stage for what Roy Porter referred to as a 'pharmacological transformation', with the pharmacist and the physician now being armed with potent medicaments for the relief of pain.

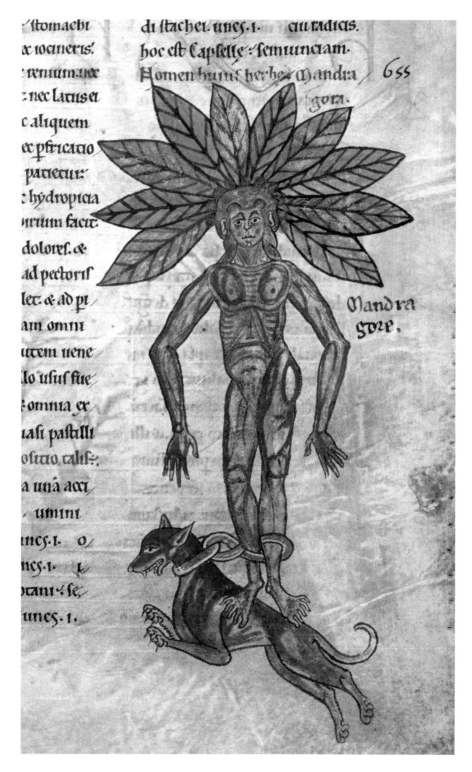

Mandrake (Mandragora Root) (c 1175). Mosan mediaeval illuminated manuscript. *London, The British Library. Harley, MS 1585, f57.* By permission of The British Library..

8

Surgery for Haemorrhoids, Nose Polyps, and Corneal Incision (c 1190–1200)

Anglo-Norman illuminated manuscript

From earliest times in the Christian West, the care of the sick was often based on monastic and other religious communities. In England they included, for example, St Bartholomew's Hospital and St Thomas' Hospital, both founded in the 12th century. Around the time this illuminated manuscript was produced, several important universities were founded: Salerno, followed by Paris in the early 12th century, Bologna (1158), Oxford (1167), Montpellier (1181), Cambridge (1209) and Padua (1222). Most practitioners might have trained at one of these centres or been apprenticed to someone who had. Furthermore, this corresponds to the period when physicians, with their concentration on herbal remedies, were separating from the surgeons. The latter became involved in dealing with the results of injuries, including reducing dislocations and treating wounds. But more often their skills were required in a number of minor surgical operations, such as cutting for the stone, tooth pulling and, as here, treating haemorrhoids, nasal polyps and cataracts.

In the case of haemorrhoids, the surgeon uses a clawed separator in his left hand while incising with his right (note that the patient stands in the bowl intended to catch the blood that is pouring over the surgeon's left knee!). In extirpating nasal polyps, the surgeon holds a knife in one hand and a pipe in the other through which to blow a healing powder. Here, the patient holds a bowl to catch the blood. Finally, the surgeon is seen treating cataracts, a technique dating back to Ayurvedic medicine and even mentioned in the Hammurabi Code in 2250 BC. According to ancient theory, cataracts were formed by a whitish liquid descending from the brain. With a long needle, the lens was displaced out of the line of vision, so-called 'couching'. All of these procedures were refined and improved over the following centuries.

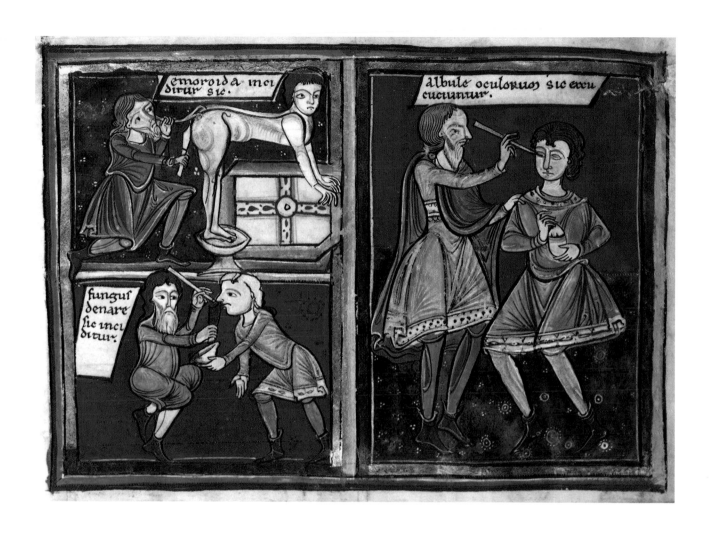

Surgery for Haemorrhoids, Nose Polyps, and Corneal Incision (c 1190–1200). Anglo-Norman illuminated manuscript. Pigments on vellum, 19.7 cm × 30 cm. *London. The British Library. Sloane, MS 1975, f93.*
By permission of The British Library.

9

Consultations Between Doctor and Patient (14th century)

Mediaeval illuminated manuscript

Before the advent of printing in the 15th century, making copies of book illustrations involved the laborious process of repeating hand-drawn works, usually carried out by monks. These have a particular interest to the medical profession when they illustrate the relationship between doctor and patient, as in this case. This shows 4 out of 48 scenes in the preface to a 14th century book of medicinal simples, or herbal remedies, by Matthew Platearius. In fact, herbal plants were often cultivated in monastery gardens. The first apothecary shop opened in London in 1345.

At the time, diagnosing a patient's condition depended on little more than uroscopy and pulse-taking. Here we see the physician's consultation concerning patients' symptoms. The top left illustration shows a patient vomiting, the top right illustration shows a patient fainting (perhaps epilepsy) and in the bottom right a patient points to his hair, which appears different from the hair of others portrayed in the series.

The bottom left illustration is particularly interesting. The patient is opening his mouth to show his teeth and presumably has toothache. Tooth extraction was seen as falling into the surgeon's field of expertise and at the time physicians tended to look down upon surgeons and their craft. This is clearly expressed here with the surgeon wearing merely a cap and arm-less gown compared with the fine robes of the trained doctor of physic! Other illustrations in the book depict nose-bleeds and rashes, etc. All illustrate patients' complaints, but there are no indications of any approaches to treatment.

It would be a long time before patients' symptoms would be associated with relevant clinical signs leading to specific diagnoses. Interestingly, this manuscript was produced in an Amiens workshop in the *early* 14th century and therefore presumably before the plague reached France in 1348/49. This would have a devastating effect on the general population and also, because physicians and surgeons became fewer in number, they would become more valued.

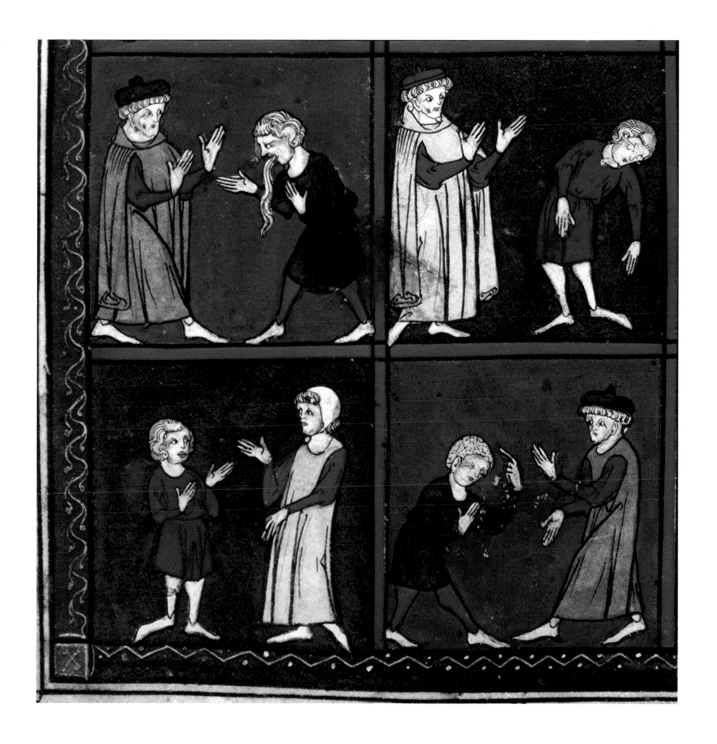

Consultations Between Doctor and Patient (14th century). Mediaeval illuminated manuscript. *London, The British Library. Sloane, MS 1977, f50v.*
By permission of The British Library.

10

Ship of Fools (c 1490–1500)

by Hieronymus Bosch

Hieronymus Bosch (c 1490–1516) was without doubt one of the most imaginative and interesting of Netherlandish painters in mediaeval times. Bosch was named after a town in Northern Brabant, where he was born and lived, and was an orthodox Catholic and a prominent member of a local religious brotherhood. His work was certainly unconventional, however, with elements of fantasy, so that later some considered him a heretic. Many of his works emphasize the greed, gluttony and folly of human beings and the fearful consequences.

In the *Ship of Fools*, Bosch depicts the consequences of foolish behaviour. At the time, the image of a ship with fools would have been very familiar to contemporaries, for in carnival processions boats filled with fools would be pulled on wheels through the streets. The symbol of a fluttering pennant with a crescent moon emphasized madness. Those in the boat do not know right from wrong. Thus the monk and nun, instead of living separately, share a meal and enjoyment together with suggestions of gluttony. The individual in a fool's costume would have been seen as merely eccentric. All the rest are behaving badly and therefore sinning against the teachings of the Church. It has even been suggested, therefore, that the work brought together two different interpretations of the fool.

The recognition of those specifically with mental illness did not emerge until much later. Admittedly, some were occasionally cared for in monasteries and similar establishments throughout Europe. In England, however, the mentally ill were often regarded as comical, as witnessed in Hogarth's illustrations of Bedlam Hospital in his *Rake's Progress* (1735), and such spectacles for public amusement were only discontinued in 1770.

That insanity was a disease of the nervous system was taught by the Edinburgh physician William Cullen (1710–1790) and was further emphasized with the appointment of Wilhelm Griesinger (1817–1868) to the first Chair of Psychiatry and Neurology in 1865, in Berlin. From the 1950s, when lithium and other anti-depressants were introduced and later antipsychotic drugs became available, most patients could be treated and managed in the community and of course were no longer, in any way, considered a source of amusement.

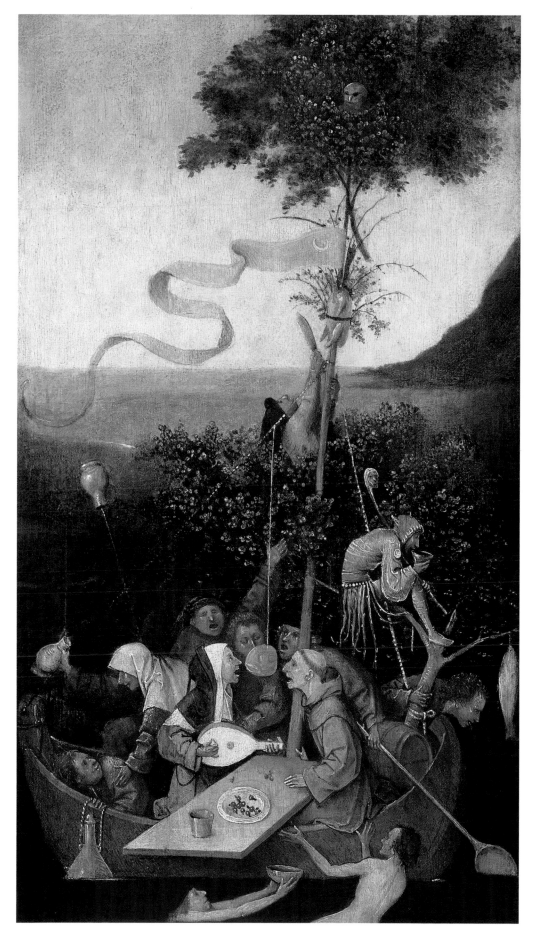

Ship of Fools (c 1490 1500) by Hieronymus Bosch. Oil on panel, 57.9 cm × 32.6 cm. *Paris, Musée du Louvre.*
© Photo RMN, © René-Gabriel Ojéda.

11

Saints Cosmas and Damian (1495)

by Alonso de Sedano

Alonso de Sedano flourished in Spain from around 1486–1530, and therefore some time after the plague that had so devastated Europe. It has been argued that as a result of the epidemic, those who survived came more to terms with their vulnerability than previously. Certainly there were many paintings afterwards that depicted suffering and death.

In Europe at this period, the Church played a prominent role in caring for the sick. In fact, certain saints became associated with healing specific diseases and some became eponymic. For example, St Vitus was associated with chorea, St Christopher with epilepsy, St Hubert with hydrophobia, St Anthony with ergotism, St Roch with bubonic plague, along with many others. Saints Cosmas and Damian were considered protectors against sickness. According to legend, the twin brothers were purported, as shown here, to have once amputated a diseased leg and grafted on the stump the leg of a Moor. With Christian persecution under the emperor Diocletian, the two saints were believed to have survived drowning, crucifixion and burning, but were finally beheaded in northern Syria in AD 303.

Besides this painting, there are several others portraying the two saints, including works by Andrea Mantegna, Francesco Pesellino, Paulo Bontulli and Hans von Kulmbach, all from around the same period in the 15th and early 16th centuries. Cosmas and Damian continued to be protectors against sickness for many years, and even today they form part of the Coat of Arms of the Royal Society of Medicine.

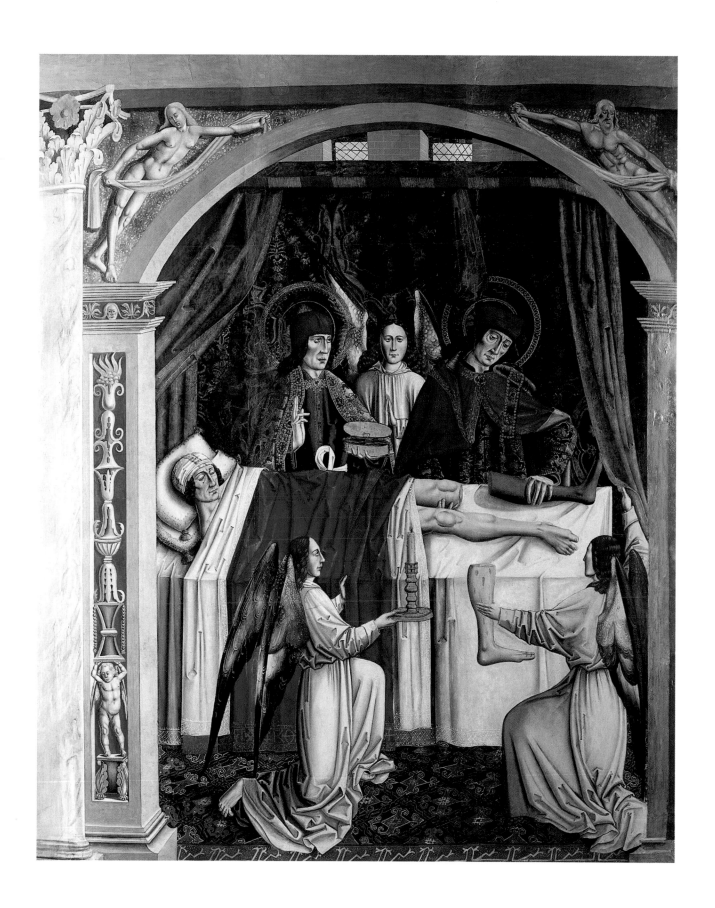

Saints Cosmas and Damian (1495) by Alonso de Sedano. Oil on wood, 169 cm × 133 cm. *London, Wellcome Library.*

12

Coat of Arms of the
Royal Society of Medicine (1927)

by Martin Travers

The Coat of Arms of the Royal Society of Medicine was designed by Martin Travers in 1927 and employs several significant medical and surgical references. The two supporting figures on either side are Saints Cosmas and Damian, considered since the 4th century to protect against sickness. The divisions of the shield into green and red represent physicians and surgeons, and thus the saint on the left holds an apothecary jar, while the saint on the right holds a scalpel. The legendary Greek god Asklepios, also associated with healing, is usually identified by a caduceus or staff entwined with a snake, and this too is portrayed against the shield.

Above is a flowering plant, which has been referred to as the herb 'all-heal'. This term has been used in the past for a variety of plants. The arrangement of the flowering head very much resembles an Umbellifer. This is a notoriously difficult group for anyone other than an expert botanist to identify. Some members of this group, such as hemlock, are poisonous! But among the Umbellifers, in view of the whitish flowers and leaf shape, it is possible that this is *sanicle*. This plant has been used from earliest times for healing. Early herbalists recommended its use for such ailments as sore throats and mouth ulcers. In the Middle Ages, it was commonly believed that 'he who keeps sanicle has no business with a doctor'.

The motto on the Coat of Arms is from Martial (*Epigrams*), 'Non est vivere sed valere vita', or, as the recent *History of the Royal Society of Medicine* by Penelope Hunting has it, 'it is important to enjoy good health to live fully'.

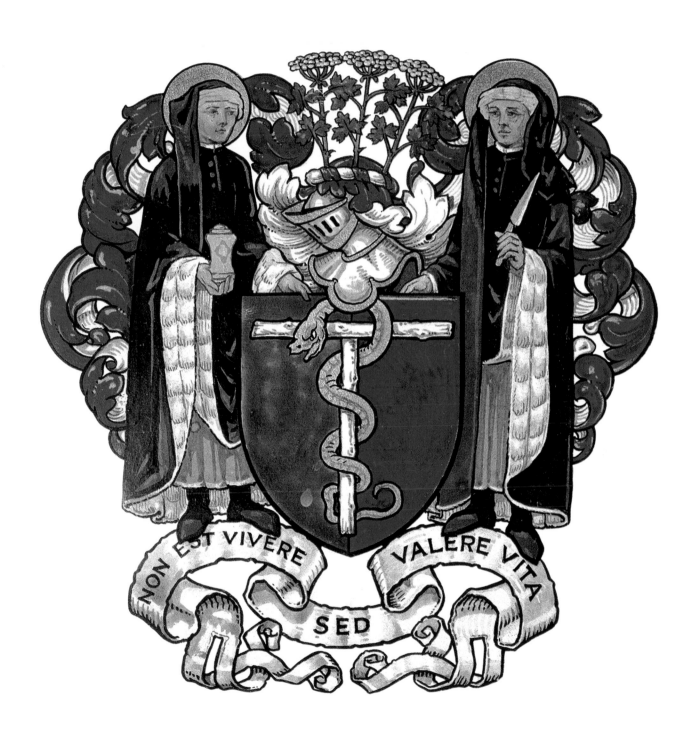

Coat of Arms of the Royal Society of Medicine (1927) by Martin Travers. *London, Royal Society of Medicine Archives.*

13

Battlefield Surgery (1465)

illuminated manuscript for Philip the Good, Duke of Burgundy

At Agincourt in 1415, the English archers with their longbows inflicted terrible injuries on the French. But it was the use of firearms, a little earlier at the battle of Crécy, that increased the range and severity of injuries. Guthrie has commented that war has always been a great teacher of surgery and that the leading surgeons of this period, as well as later, were army surgeons. Although advances were made, major innovations in the subject did not occur until the 19th century. Nevertheless, there were some very notable surgeons who demonstrated considerable skills, such as Ambroise Paré (1510–1590) of France, who is considered to be the greatest surgeon of the Renaissance and who practised as an army surgeon during the period when firearms had been introduced. He is credited with abandoning the cauterization and boiling oil treatment of gunshot wounds in favour of a gently acting balm and salve. He also introduced the use of ligating blood vessels in performing amputations. He frequently remarked 'Je le pansait; Dieu le guarit' in Old French, meaning 'I dressed the wound, God healed him'.

This was the period when the physicians and surgeons began to go their separate ways. In England, the Surgeon's Guild and the Barber's Company were formally united as Barber-Surgeons by an Act of Parliament in 1540. But many Barber-Surgeons not only carried out surgical procedures, but also became engaged in 'physic', treating for example venereal disease, often using mercurial compounds.

This illustration from an illuminated manuscript of 1465 is of the siege of a city by Hannibal and the Carthaginians. But the event would actually have been part of the Second Punic War in the 2nd century BC. However, the artist is depicting a battle scene and surgery as it was in the 15th century. The surgeon deals with a wounded soldier in a tent reserved for the purpose. He is dressing a leg wound and has several vessels and jars at his disposal that would have contained various medicaments. This manuscript was written and illuminated for Philip the Good (1396–1467), the Duke of Burgundy, who was a powerful military leader and committed Crusader at the time.

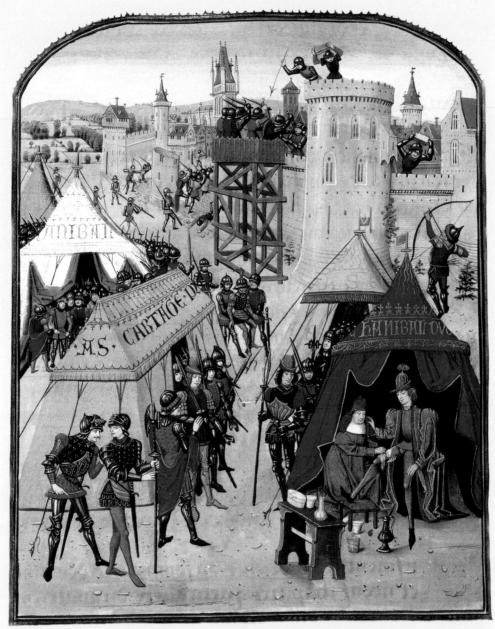

14

St Elizabeth Tending the Sick (c 1597)

by Adam Elsheimer

Much of the care of the sick, until relatively recently, fell to the responsibility of organizations dependent on the Church and monasteries. Here, the German artist Adam Elsheimer (1578–1610) depicts a scene of St Elizabeth tending the sick as he imagined it some 400 years earlier. She was born in 1207, the daughter of the Hungarian King Andreas II, and at the age of 14 married Ludwig IV of Thuringia, but she was widowed at the age of 20 with three children. She refused to remarry, renounced all her privileges, left her children and went to Marburg to found a small hospital for the care of the sick. She died in 1231 at the age of 24 and was later canonized.

Despite the small size of this work, it includes much noteworthy detail. In the foreground, St Elizabeth tends a patient in bed, and her Coat of Arms is mounted above the window. The religious basis of the hospital is evident from the statue of the Madonna and Child on the far wall.

The artist may have intended the man with the red hat to represent a trained physician although in fact there were very few such individuals in the 13th century. Most therapy would have centred on herbal remedies. Uroscopy played a major role in diagnosis, and there are urine flasks on a side table on the left and below the statue of the Madonna. Leprosy had existed in Europe since at least the 7th century, and it has been suggested that the man on the right with a bandaged leg may have had the disease – although this is purely speculation.

Elsheimer produced many other delightful and well-crafted works, which were later acclaimed by, for example, Rubens. But he died in poverty at the early age of 32.

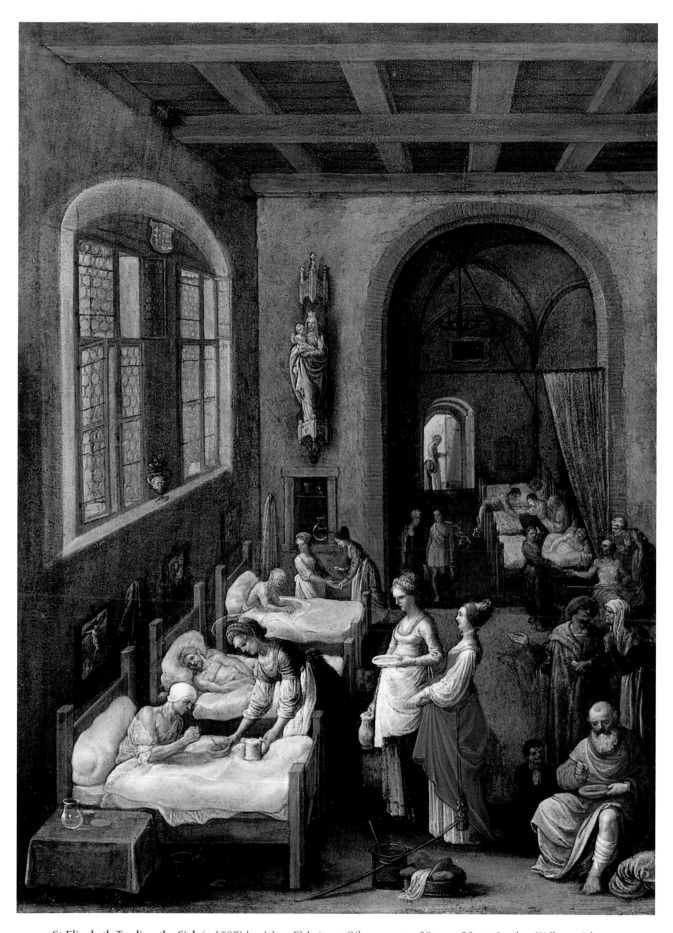

St Elizabeth Tending the Sick (c 1597) by Adam Elsheimer. Oil on copper, 28 cm × 20 cm. *London, Wellcome Library.*

15

Seven Acts of Charity: Visiting the Sick (1504)
by the Master of Alkmaar

The Master of Alkmaar is so named after the altarpiece of the *Seven Works of Mercy*, painted in 1504 for the Church of St Lawrence (Laurenskerk) in Alkmaar. The artist may have been Cornelis Buys. At the end of the First World War, the seven panels were transferred to the Rijksmuseum in Amsterdam.

The *Seven Mercies* comprise feeding the hungry, refreshing the thirsty, clothing the naked, burying the dead, lodging the traveller, nursing the sick and finally, comforting prisoners. Each bears an exhortation to the observer. A very similar work by Michael Sweerts (1618–1664), another Flemish painter, is entitled *The Seven Works of Charity*. In both of these works, the object was to represent everyday occurrences peopled by individuals in everyday dress, with whom the observer could identify. The emphasis was on the need for pity, and praise for those who did good. The rather cheerless colour has been said to help emphasize the puritanical background. The emphasis was on an active form of Christianity that was a major feature in caring for the sick at the time and continued until comparatively recently.

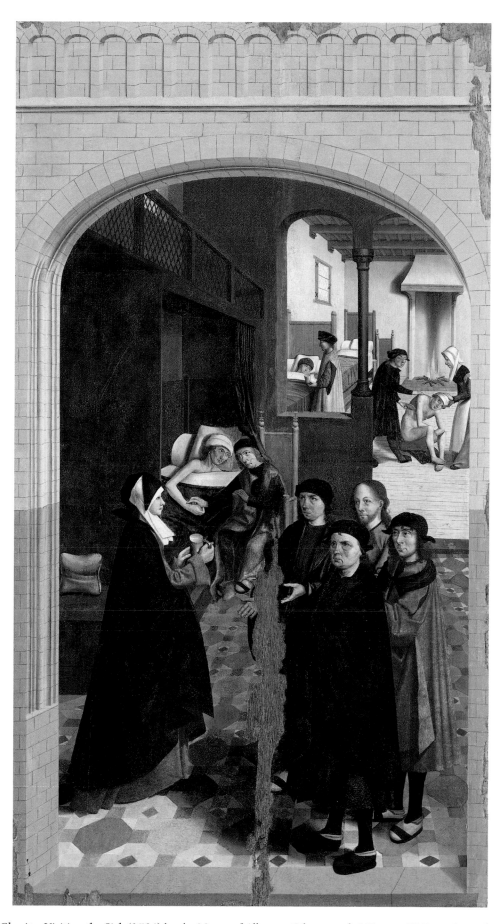

Seven Acts of Charity: Visiting the Sick (1504) by the Master of Alkmaar. Oil on panel, 101 cm × 55.5 cm. *Amsterdam, Rijksmuseum.*

16

Anatomical Drawings: Myology of Trunk (c 1509–1510)

by Leonardo da Vinci

The early history of human anatomical studies begins in Greece with Herophilus (c 350–280 BC) and Erasistratus (c 310–250 BC), who are credited as being the first to study the structures of the human body from dissected corpses. Their writings, however, were lost – reference to them is through the works of another Greek, Galen (c AD 130–200). Galen was a renowned physician and anatomist who wrote extensively – more than 130 of his works have survived. For a period, he was chief physician to the gladiators at Pergamum, the city of his birth, but spent most of his life in Rome. He was an expert dissector, but by this time dissection had lost support from the authorities and most of his studies were therefore based on animals. This led to errors that were perpetuated for many centuries through reference to his works. For example, he described a network of blood vessels at the base of the brain that, although present in some animals, is absent in humans. Nevertheless, he did make a number of important observations: that many muscles are arranged in antagonistic pairs, that there are seven pairs of cranial nerves, and that there is a distinction between arteries and veins.

Because of the prohibition of dissection, the distinguished Arabian surgeon Albucasis (926–1013), then in Cordoba, was forced to conclude that the reason surgery as a speciality had almost completely disappeared from Spain was because of a lack of good anatomical knowledge. Nevertheless, by the 13th century, a limited number of human dissections were being carried out by a number of eminent anatomists, such as Mondino de Luzzi in Bologna and later Henri de Mondeville (c 1270–1320) in Montpellier. By the 15th century however, the restrictions on human dissection had been gradually relaxed. It was at this point that Leonardo da Vinci (1452–1519) produced his sketch books, in which he collaborated with the anatomist Marc Antonio della Torre, who taught at Padua and Parvia. Leonardo's anatomical drawings were based on some 30 dissections. These are also detailed in his attached notes, written backwards. Not only were his drawings of considerable artistic merit in their own right, but they also revealed that Leonardo had made several important anatomical discoveries: for example the maxillary sinus, the ventricles of the brain and the membranes covering the foetus in utero. William Hunter, the surgeon, when he first saw the originals in King George III's library at Windsor commented:

'When I consider what pains he has taken upon every part of the body, the superiority of his universal genius, his particular excellence in mechanics and hydraulics, and the attention with which such a man would examine and see objects which he has to draw, I am fully persuaded that Leonardo was the best Anatomist, at that time, in the world...' (Letter, 1784).

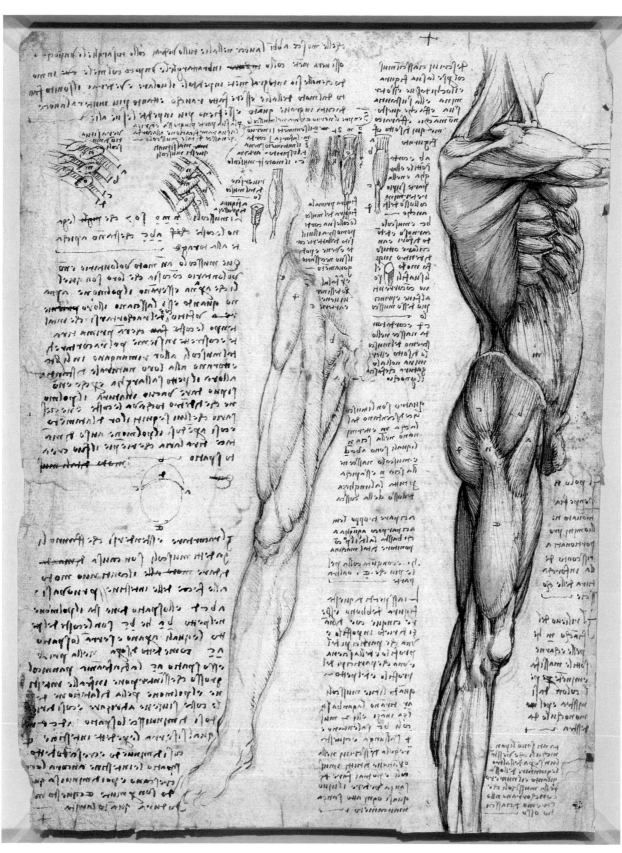

Anatomical Drawings: Myology of Trunk (c 1509–1510) by Leonardo da Vinci. Pen and ink. *Windsor, Royal Collection.*
The Royal Collection © 2005, Her Majesty Queen Elizabeth II.

17

Portrait of Vesalius Teaching Anatomy, Aged 28 (1543)

anonymous

Many eminent historians, including most recently John Gribbin, date the beginning of the scientific reformation in Europe to 1543. This was the year the Polish astronomer Nicolaus Copernicus died and his book, *De Revolutionibus Orbium Coelestium* (*The Revolution of Celestial Spheres*) was published, in which he suggested that the Earth was not the centre of the universe but that it was merely a planet orbiting the Sun. In the same year, one of the major landmarks in biological, and in particular medical, science was published, namely *De Humani Corporis Fabrica* (*The Structure of the Human Body*) by Andreas Vesalius (1514–1564). Vesalius was born in Brussels of a well-known medical family, his father being an apothecary. He was educated at the University of Louvain and later went to Paris to study medicine, where he met another Belgian, Jan Stefan van Calcar (or Kalkar). The latter was a pupil of Titian and later is believed to have been responsible for the excellent illustrations that adorn the anatomical works of Vesalius, perhaps including this portrait of him. Recent research, however, indicates that some other students may have been involved, even Vesalius himself.

In 1537, Vesalius was appointed Professor of Surgery and Anatomy at Padua, and it was in this capacity that he produced his magnificent opus. In the course of his human dissections he found that many of the anatomical teachings at the time were in error, being based on the much earlier work of Galen, who had centred most of his work on animal dissections. For example, the human liver had two, not five, lobes, the sternum had three, not seven, parts, the mandible was a single bone, and, most importantly, there was no direct communication between the two cardiac ventricles. When Vesalius' magnum opus was published exposing these errors by the previously much-revered Galen, he attracted much criticism and animosity, which forced him to resign his Chair. He left for Madrid to become a physician to the nobility. His revolutionary anatomical studies had been crowded into three short years and were now over. For reasons that are not entirely clear, he went on a pilgrimage to Jerusalem and died on the Greek island of Zante on the return journey. He had made anatomy a science – and all future developments in surgery would always be indebted to his work.

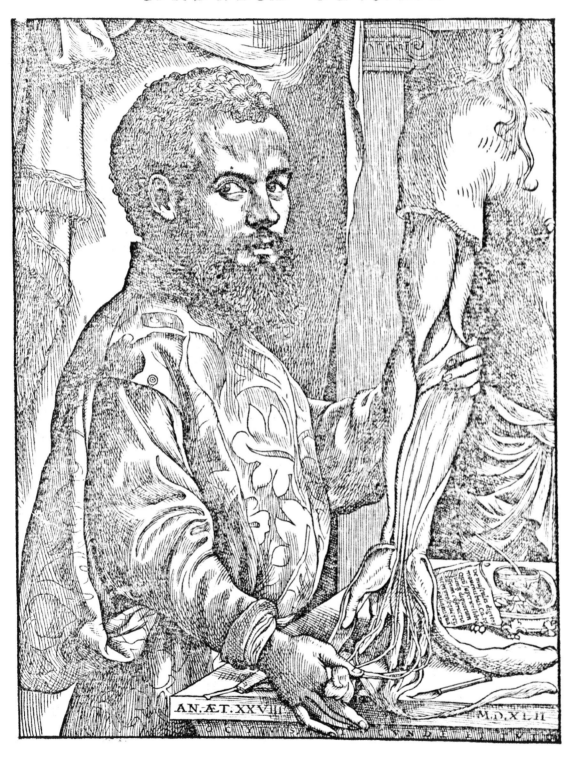

Portrait of Andreas Vesalius Teaching Anatomy, Aged 28 (1543), anonymous, from the Frontispiece of *De Humani Corporis Fabrica.*
Woodcut. *London, Royal Society of Medicine Library.*

18

The Anatomy Lecture of Dr Joan Deyman (1656)

by Rembrandt van Rijn

Rembrandt (1606–1669) has been considered the greatest of all Dutch painters. Apart from his obvious artistic merit and superb craftsmanship, some of his work is of special interest to physicians and surgeons in a number of ways. For example, he created no less than 86 self-portraits from the age of 15 until the year of his death, revealing in telling detail the facial changes associated with aging. Furthermore, his painting *Bathsheba with King David's Letter* (1654) has attracted attention because some believe the apparent distortion of the left breast of the model, Hendrickje Stoffels, Rembrandt's mistress, could have been due to breast cancer. But this seems unlikely because, without treatment, she nevertheless survived a further nine years.

Perhaps of greater medical interest are those Rembrandt works concerned with public dissections and anatomy teaching, including *The Anatomy Lesson of Dr Tulp* (1632), which was Rembrandt's first major success, and this painting of Dr Joan Deyman. Dr Tulp or Tulpius (1593–1674) was a professor in Amsterdam and was regarded as one of the greatest anatomists of his time. Most students of anatomy, however, draw attention to the fact that in the painting, the artist appears to have the flexors of the fingers arising from the lateral epicondyle of the humerus and not the medial epicondyle!

In this painting, Dr Joan (Johan) Deyman is seen deflecting the scalp and removing the cranium to expose the brain. Deyman (1620–1666) had succeeded Tulp as prelector of the Surgeon's Guild three years before this painting. As in the work of Dr Tulp, the subject was a condemned criminal. In this case he was executed on 28 January 1656 and dissected over the following three or four days. This was important because the cold winter weather would prevent excessive putrefaction. Incidentally, the original painting was larger but was cut down after being damaged by fire some 67 years later. Apart from its medical aspects, the work is also of interest because of the foreshortening of the corpse. It is reminiscent of Andrea Mantegna's *The Dead Christ* (c 1501) and reflects a growing concern among artists with attempts to represent subjects in a three-dimensional perspective. This interest had been developing since the 15th century in the work of artists such as Uccello and Piero della Francesca.

By the time this work was created, human dissection as a means of teaching anatomy was becoming accepted, particularly in Italy, Holland and France and, to a lesser extent, in Germany. In Britain, anatomy teaching became firmly established as an academic discipline in Edinburgh Medical School with the three generations of the Monros, beginning with Alexander Monro *primus* from 1720. The subject gained increasing acceptance, but the acquisition of bodies for dissection often proved a problem with the emergence of 'grave robbers' and 'resurrectionists'. The Anatomy Act was passed in 1832 in order to legitimize the practice, and Gray's celebrated anatomy textbook first appeared some years later in 1858.

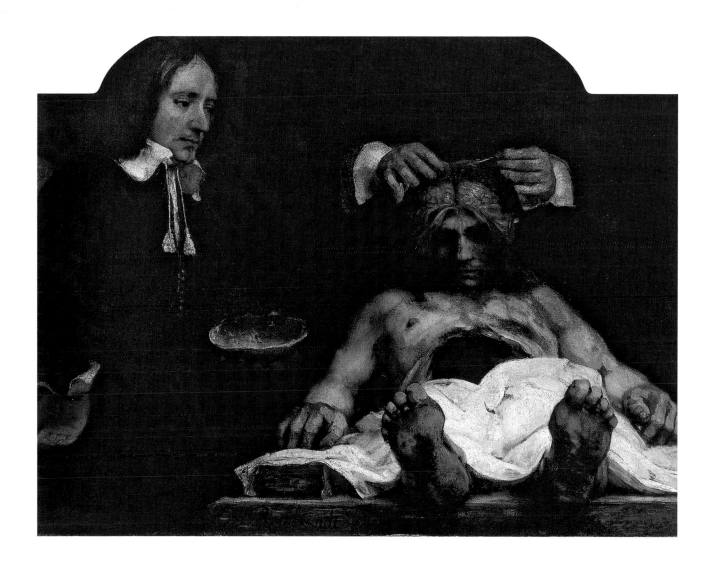

The Anatomy Lecture of Dr Joan Deyman (1656) by Rembrandt van Rijn. Oil on canvas, 100 cm × 134 cm. *Amsterdam, Amsterdams Historisch Museum.*

19

The Fountain of Youth (1546)

by Lucas Cranach the Elder

This work by the German painter Lucas Cranach the Elder (1472–1553), painted in 1546, depicts the scene of a public bath. Although partly of course a product of the artist's imagination, baths like this did exist in such places as Vichy and Baden Baden and were popular throughout the Middle Ages, the waters being believed to have powers of rejuvenation and miraculous cures. Here, Cranach imagines a spring that could restore bathers to their youth. We see old ladies entering the pool on the left, to emerge as young maidens on the right to meet well-dressed young men, who then dine, dance and carouse together. It could be of significance that Cranach was 74 when he painted this scene and perhaps hoped for similar rejuvenation! But some of the bathers are clearly ill, being brought to the spring in carts and stretchers. A doctor in his red robe on the left appears to be examining such a person.

In England by the 18th century, spas flourished in such places as Bath, Tunbridge Wells, Buxton, Scarborough, Malvern and Cheltenham. They were promoted as centres for health through abstinence and dietary restrictions, which were worthy ambitions since many visiting the spas were overweight and frequently suffered from gout. But they also became centres for social gatherings, including assignations, and 'taking the waters' was often satirized by artists such as Thomas Rowlandson and writers such as Tobias Smollett. They also attracted many charlatans and quacks who promoted their special diets and potions. One such was Dr William Oliver FRS, who advocated his particular brand of biscuit, which is still sold today as 'Bath Olivers'.

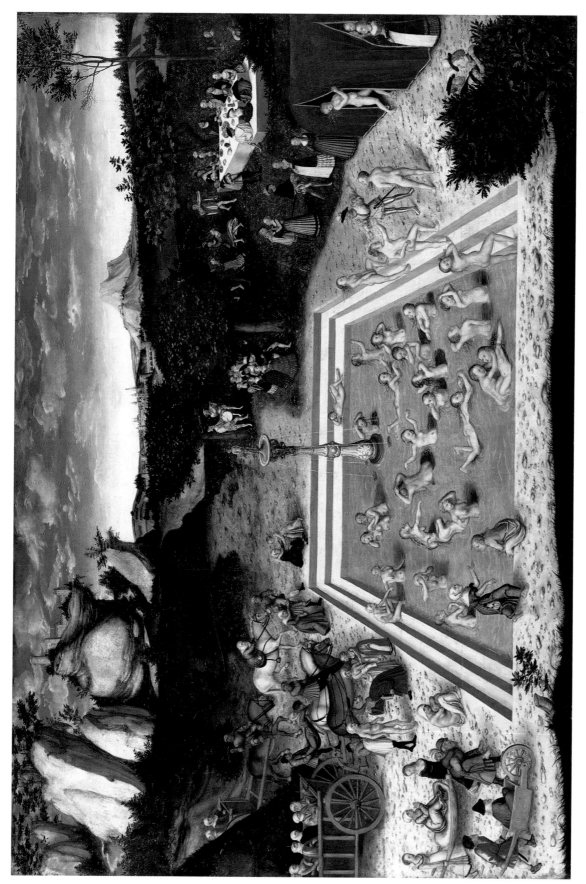

The Fountain of Youth (1546) by Lucas Cranach the Elder. Oil on wood, 121 cm × 184 cm. Berlin, Gemäldegalerie, Staatliche Museen zu Berlin.
© Bildarchiv Preussicher Kulturbesitz, Berlin, 2005. Photo: Joerg P. Anders.

20

Short-Robed Surgeon Catheterises a Patient (c 1510)

anonymous, after Heinrich Füllmaurer and Albrecht Meyer

In this work the surgeon is catheterizing a man to relieve urinary obstruction. This might have been the result of a urinary stricture secondary to, for example, a venereal infection. A variety of catheters and bougies were developed for this purpose. But perhaps more likely is that urinary obstruction resulted from stones or 'gravel'.

The surgical treatment of bladder stones dates back to the earliest times. It is mentioned, for example, in the Oath of Hippocrates (c 460–370 BC). The Roman Celsus (25 BC – AD 50) gave an excellent description of perineal lithotomy in the 1st century, whereby the surgeon cut down on to the base of the bladder, through the perineum to remove the stone. Before anaesthesia, the pain must have been virtually unbearable. The patient was held down firmly by several assistants and the aim was to complete the procedure as quickly as possible, often in only a minute or two.

Another approach involved dilating the urethra and extracting the stone, or passing crushing instruments into the bladder along the urethra – so-called transurethral lithotomy. Because of the difficulties and dangers of cutting for the stone, it was natural that this was the favoured method by many, and a great variety of lithotrites were developed for the purpose.

Yet another approach was to open the bladder directly through an incision in the lower abdomen: suprapubic lithotomy or the 'high operation'. But this was fraught with problems and dangers, and did not find favour until the 18th century – largely through the success of William Cheselden (1688–1752), the celebrated London surgeon.

Incidentally, in this watercolour the surgeon wears a short robe denoting that he was a travelling barber-surgeon who did various minor surgical procedures, as distinct from 'gentlemen of the long robe', trained and licensed to practice all manner of surgical procedures.

Bladder stones were very common among infants as well as adults and were not infrequent until the end of the 19th century. The explanation is not entirely clear. But, as Harold Ellis has noted, bladder stones with accompanying discomfort affected such luminaries as Francis Bacon, Isaac Newton, William Harvey, Oliver Cromwell and Samuel Pepys. It is interesting to speculate how this distressing condition influenced their work.

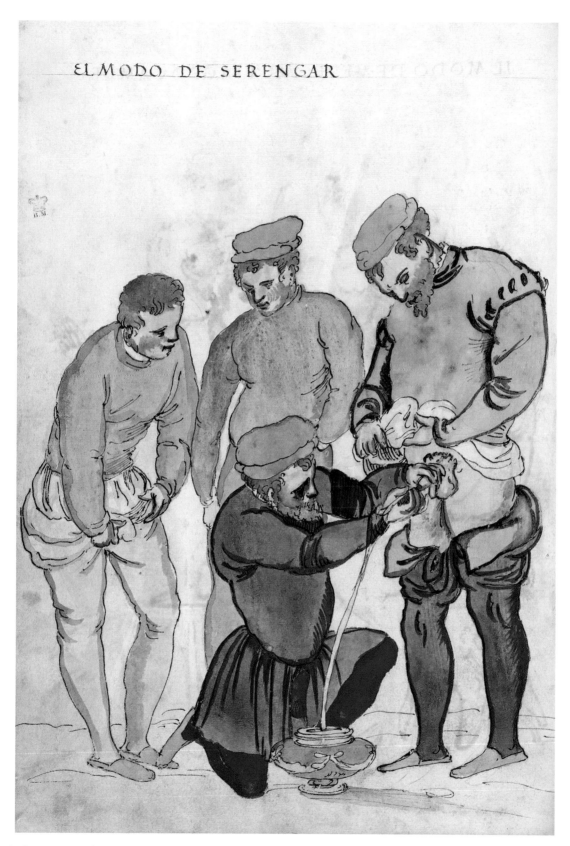

Short-Robed Surgeon Catheterizes a Patient (c 1510) anonymous, after Heinrich Füllmaurer and Albrecht Meyer. Illustration from *Sketchbook*. Pen and ink and watercolour, 41.8 cm × 27 cm. *London, British Museum. 1928–3–10–94.*
© Copyright of the Trustees of the British Museum.

21

Three Miniatures:
Henry Fitzroy, Duke of Richmond
(c 1533–1535)
by Lucas Horenbout

Henry Brandon, 2nd Duke of Suffolk (c 1541)
Charles Brandon, 3rd Duke of Suffolk (c 1541)
by Hans Holbein the Younger

These three works of art illustrate the beginnings of miniature portrait painting in England. Lucas Horenbout (or Luke Hornebolt) grew up in Flanders, the son of a Court painter. The family, however, moved to England to escape persecution for their Lutheran sympathies in the 1520s. Horenbout rapidly rose to fame and was held in high regard in the court of Henry VIII for his miniature painting, and was granted the title of 'King's Painter' in 1534. He is generally accepted as the originator of miniature painting in England. He died in 1544.

Hans Holbein the Younger (c 1497–1543) was trained by his father and was active first in Germany and later in Switzerland and then England, where he died from the plague in 1543. He also became famed for his miniature painting, having learnt the art from Horenbout, and was later to be followed by another equally famous limner, Nicholas Hilliard.

Apart from the obvious artistic merit of these beautifully executed miniatures, they are also of interest from a medical point of view. Henry Fitzroy (1519–1536) was the illegitimate son of Henry VIII. He died of tuberculosis a year or so after this painting was executed. The disease, however, had already begun to take its toll, as witnessed by the unusual dress of nightcap and shift in which the subject is depicted.

Henry Brandon and his younger brother were renowned scholars, but in their teens, in 1541, both fell ill from the 'sweating sickness' and died within half an hour of each other. This was an acute illness quite different from the more chronic condition that afflicted Henry Fitzroy. But the precise nature of the 'sweating illness' or 'English sweat' is debatable and one of the great puzzles of historical epidemiology. It was first noted around 1485 and was characterized by a sudden acute fever with profuse sweating. It mainly affected young men among the economically advantaged, and victims usually succumbed within 24–48 hours. It has been variously attributed to a possible virus (even an arbovirus) or toxin (including ergot). But these ideas are purely speculative. It has been argued that English methods of therapy, which encouraged perspiration and purgation, may have exacerbated fluid and salt loss and thus led to circulatory collapse. Whatever the cause of the demise of the three subjects of these paintings, clearly their memory lives on in these beautifully executed miniatures.

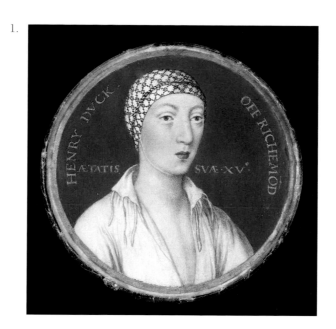

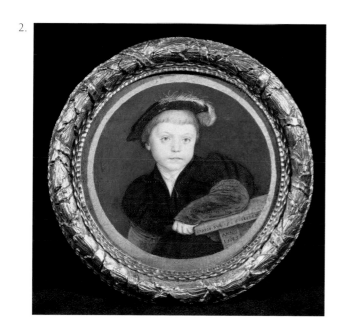

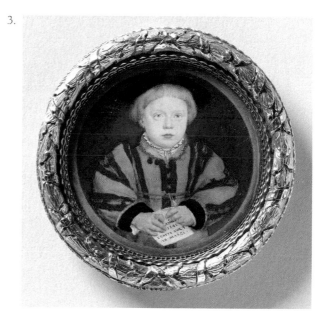

1. **Henry Fitzroy, Duke of Richmond** (c 1533–1535) by Lucas Horenbout. Watercolour on vellum laid on playing card (the ace of hearts), diameter 44 mm.

2. **Henry Brandon, 2nd Duke of Suffolk** (c 1541) by Hans Holbein the Younger. Vellum laid on playing card (the king of a suit), diameter 56 mm.

3. **Charles Brandon, 3rd Duke of Suffolk** (c 1541) by Hans Holbein the Younger. Vellum laid on playing card (the ace of clubs), diameter 55 mm.

Windsor, Royal Collection.

The Royal Collection © 2005, Her Majesty Queen Elizabeth II.

22

Henry VIII in 1540 Handing to Thomas Vicary the Act of Union Between the Barbers and Surgeons of London (1541)

by Hans Holbein the Younger

By the time Henry VIII came to the throne of England in 1509, the distinction between surgeon and physician was being clarified, with the latter forming their own College some nine years later. The surgeons associated themselves more and more with the Barber's Company. In an Act of Parliament of 12 July 1540, the Surgeon's Guild and the Barber's Company were formally united. This act of incorporation is commemorated in this painting by Holbein the Younger (c 1497–1543), the German artist who, having settled in England, was befriended by the King. In the last 10 years of his life, Holbein completed no less than 150 portraits and scenes of the Royal Court. Here the King, sumptuously dressed and holding the Sword of State, presents the Statute to Thomas Vicary, the first surgical Master of the Company. On the left of the King kneel two of the Royal Physicians: Dr John Chambre and Dr William Butts, along with the Royal Apothecary, Thomas Alsop. William Butts was one of the physicians who attended the confinements of Anne Boleyn and later Jane Seymour.

The Barber-Surgeons Company survived for nearly 200 years until, in 1745, the surgeons formed their own separate body, eventually becoming the Royal College of Surgeons of London in 1800 and, in 1843, the Royal College of Surgeons of England. The physicians formed their own Royal College in 1851. Meanwhile, in 1815, the Apothecaries Act specified that those who were not at all medically trained should be restricted to preparing and selling medicines and thereafter referred to as druggists or pharmaceutical chemists.

In Scotland, the Incorporation of Barber-Surgeons was established in 1505 and became the Royal College of Surgeons of Edinburgh in 1778.

Incidentally, for many years, surgeons were considered inferior to physicians and hence were entitled merely 'Mr' in Britain, although apparently nowhere else.

This painting really epitomizes the very beginning of the distinct specialities of medicine, surgery and pharmacy – although in many ways the distinction nowadays is once more becoming less clear, with all three specialities often collaborating in care.

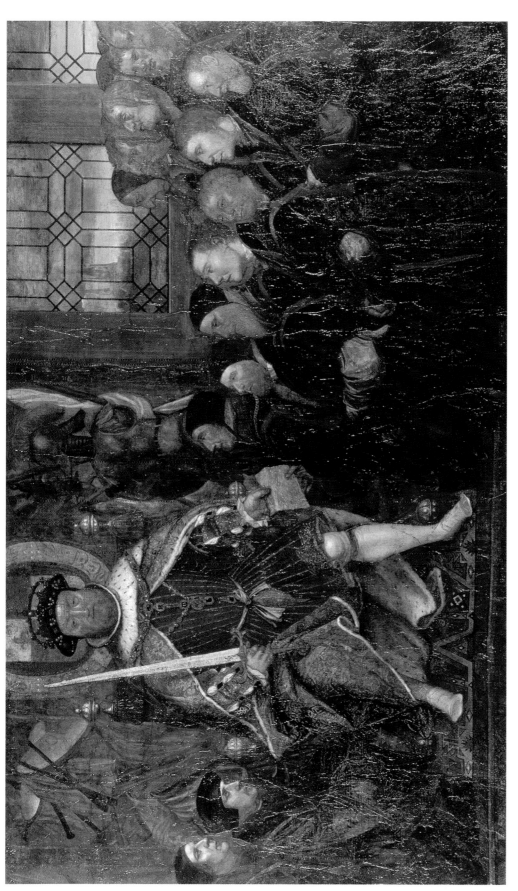

Henry VIII in 1540 Handing to Thomas Vicary the Act of Union Between the Barbers and Surgeons of London (1541) by Hans Holbein the Younger. Oil over cartoon on paper, 160 cm × 280 cm. *London, Royal College of Surgeons.*

Reproduced by kind permission of the President and Council of the Royal College of Surgeons of England.

23

Back Operation (Early 17th century)
by Adriaen Brouwer

The Flemish artist Adriaen Brouwer (1605/6–1638) was taught first by his father, a tapestry maker, and spent most of his life in Antwerp. He may have died of plague when the disease ravaged the city. He was much influenced by Bruegel and is one of the earliest genre painters in the Low Countries. He is noted particularly for his keen observation and biting humour. He clearly shared the life of the people he portrayed. He apparently made most of his quick drawings on the spot in ale houses and paid his bills with his work. In his many paintings he portrayed the low life of peasant folk and several tavern scenes with carousing, gambling and brawling. His *Bitter Draught* illustrates in a very graphic way the response to taking an unpalatable medicine. His work was eagerly collected by both Rubens and Rembrandt.

Several of his works are particularly interesting from a surgical point of view. In one he shows an itinerant barber-surgeon performing a foot operation, in another an operation on the arm. He also painted two instances of a back operation, as here. This may have been some form of skin tumour, but more likely was a boil or carbuncle. Such skin infections were very common in the past. With poor hygiene, deep-seated infections would develop, involving the entire hair follicle and subcutaneous tissues. The most common sites would have been parts exposed to irritation, friction, and moisture, such as the back. Although nowadays these infections are usually due to *Staphylococcus aureus*, in the past, among those working in agriculture, the cause may also have been a mycotic infection such as sporotrichosis or even anthrax. Clearly the patient is in great pain, but may well have benefited beforehand from a tankard or two of ale.

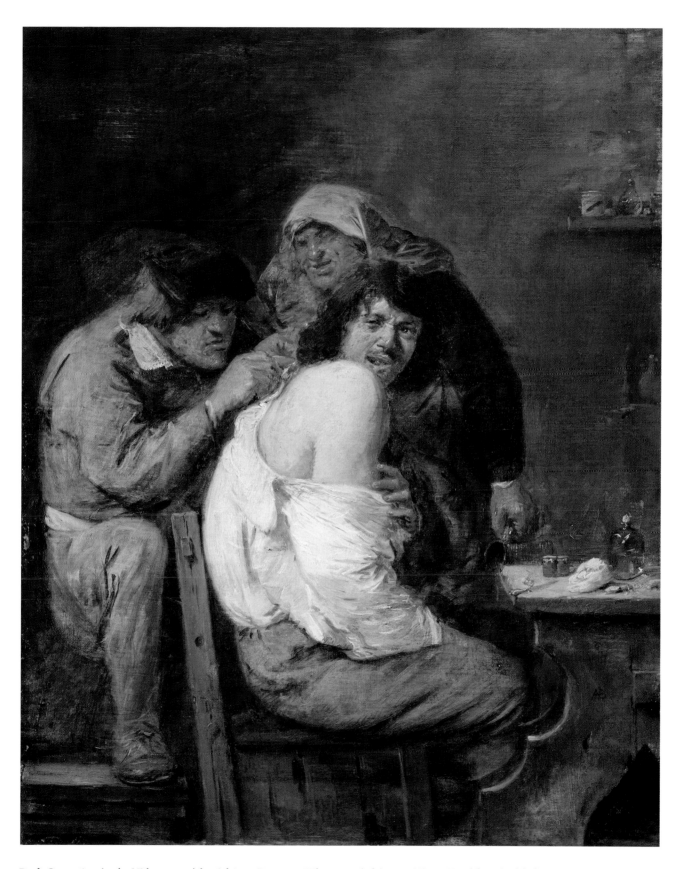

Back Operation (early 17th century) by Adriaen Brouwer. Oil on panel, 34 cm × 27 cm. *Frankfurt, Städelsches Kunstinstitut.* Photo © Kurt Haase, Artothek.

24

The Doctor's Visit (1650–1665)

by Jan Steen

Jan Steen (c 1626–1679) was one of the most prolific of Dutch painters, nearly 900 paintings having been ascribed to him. His work is interesting because much of it deals with ordinary everyday life in Dutch homes of the period – so-called genre paintings. Like several other artists at the time, he often ridiculed the profession, but in a humorous way, while at the same time pointing out the gullibility of the public. These works often rely on symbols to emphasize their meaning and would have been well recognized and appreciated by viewers at the time.

The Doctor's Visit is one of Steen's favourite themes in over 40 different versions. Here, however, a note lying on the floor declares in Dutch that no doctor is needed since this is the pain of love! Over the door is a cupid figure and on the wall hangs a painting of a pair of lovers as if to emphasize the point. The doctor is elaborately over-dressed as a character from an Italian Commedia dell'Arte and in all seriousness writes out a prescription for the young lady patient languishing in bed. The old woman in attendance shares her confidences with the doctor as to the true cause of the patient's supposed illness, while a young urchin gleefully holds a clyster aloft. This was used for rectal injections of water and other fluids and had been in general use since the 15th century for such complaints as constipation. But here it is employed by the artist in a sexual connotation. The prescription 'You are in great need of clystering' had at the time a more graphic and vulgar meaning! The use of clysters was often lampooned by many artists, such as Rowlandson, Hogarth and Cruikshank in Britain.

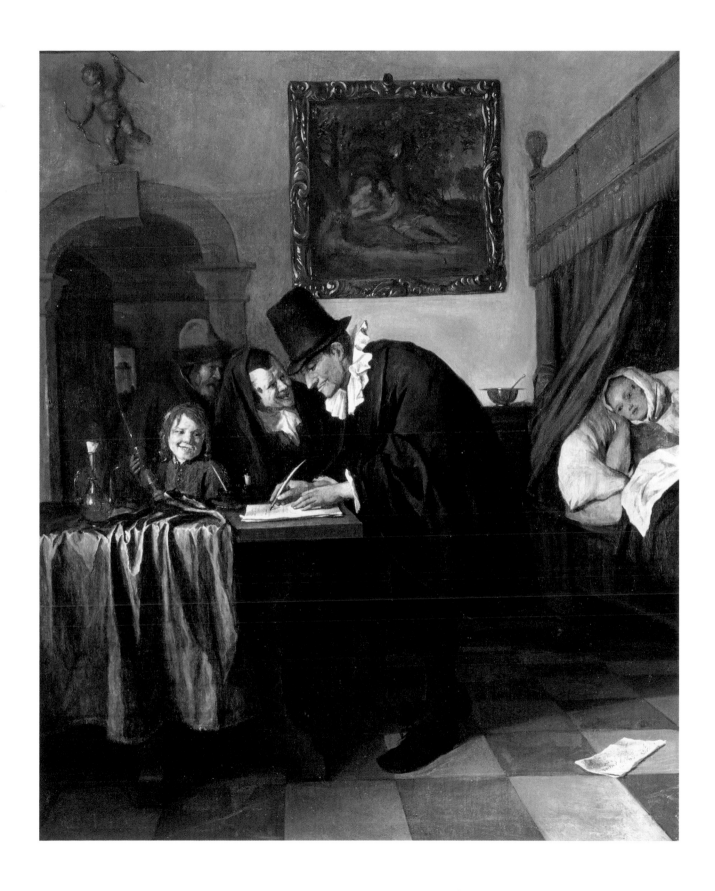

The Doctor's Visit (1650–1665) by Jan Steen. Oil on panel, 61 cm × 49.5 cm. *Rotterdam, Willem van der Vorm Foundation, Museum Boijmans Van Beuningen.*

25

The Extraction of the Stone (1650–1665)

by Jan Steen

From the time of Hippocrates, mental illness was commonly labelled either mania or melancholia, being characterized in the former by excitement and in the latter by depression, both being marked by peculiar behaviour. The theories of causation were legion, ranging from abnormalities of the bile and excesses of venery to demonic possession. The suggested treatments were also infinite. One superstition, common at the time of this painting, was that the cause was a stone in the head, and a mentally unbalanced person was often described as having 'stones' or 'rocks in the head'. Itinerant quacks took advantage of the belief by making a superficial incision in the scalp and palming a stone or stones dropped into a convenient dish held by an assistant or relative of the patient. The theme was repeated by many artists, most notably in Bosch's *Cure for Folly* (c 1480) and Bruegel the Elder's *Extraction of the Stone of Madness* (1556).

In this work of the mid 17th century by Jan Steen, some of the audience are enjoying the spectacle – although clearly not the patient himself. One wonders how these artists might have depicted some of our current practices that are of unproven and doubtful merit!

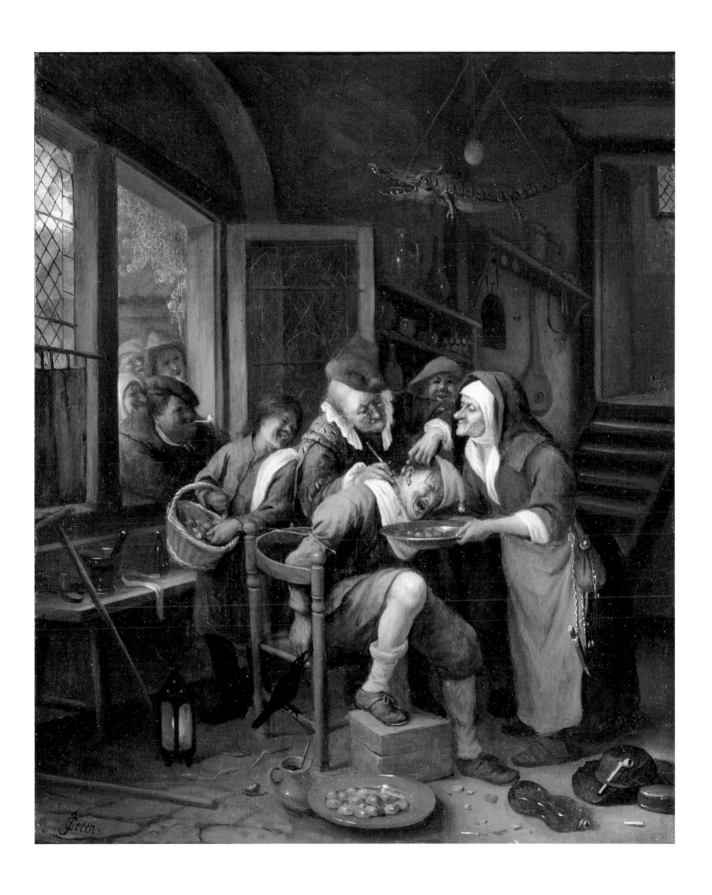

The Extraction of the Stone (1650–1665) by Jan Steen. Oil on canvas, 58.5 cm × 49 cm. *Rotterdam, Museum Boijmans Van Beuningen.*

26

The Tooth Puller (early 17th century)
by Theodor Rombouts

With no dental hygiene as we now know it, in the past dental caries must have been common. Yet there are very few instances of tooth decay and dental abscesses in Egyptian mummies until the first millennium BC, perhaps because of increasing foreign influence and dietary changes. Unfortunately, little is known about the technique of dental extraction at this time in Egypt, but there is ample evidence of tooth extraction in Western art from the 14th century, and it is often depicted, as here, in graphic detail.

Tooth extraction to a small extent fell within the province of barber-surgeons. Some very notable surgeons became distinguished in the field of dentistry, including Guy de Chauliac in the 14th century and Ambroise Paré in the 16th century. The latter even practised tooth transplantation, which in Britain was recommended by the great anatomist and surgeon John Hunter and continued until the end of the 18th century, when it was abandoned because of clinical failure, now known to be due to rejection.

Most tooth extractions in the past were carried out by itinerant tooth-pullers. They would arrive in a town on market day, when they would set up their business. Many such events were depicted by Dutch and Flemish painters of the 16th and 17th century. The tooth-puller is often surrounded by onlookers, some of whom genuinely seem to sympathize with the patient, although others seem to take delight in the spectacle: schadenfreude!

Theodor Rombouts (1579–1637) was an Antwerp painter but spent several years in Rome, coming under the influence of Caravaggio with dramatic effects produced by contrived lighting – as evident in this work. Although the tooth-puller appears to have many tools and implements to call upon, not infrequently the tooth or even the jaw would break. There was of course no anaesthesia for at least another 200 years.

It was to be a very long time before dentistry, as such, was recognized as a discipline separate from surgery. In Britain, the first dental hospital to be established was the Royal Dental Hospital of London in 1858 (later amalgamated with Guy's Hospital). Many other dental hospitals were established subsequently. But dentists were not required to be state-recognized until 1921. The specialized and sophisticated professional practice nowadays is a very far cry from the situation depicted in this work.

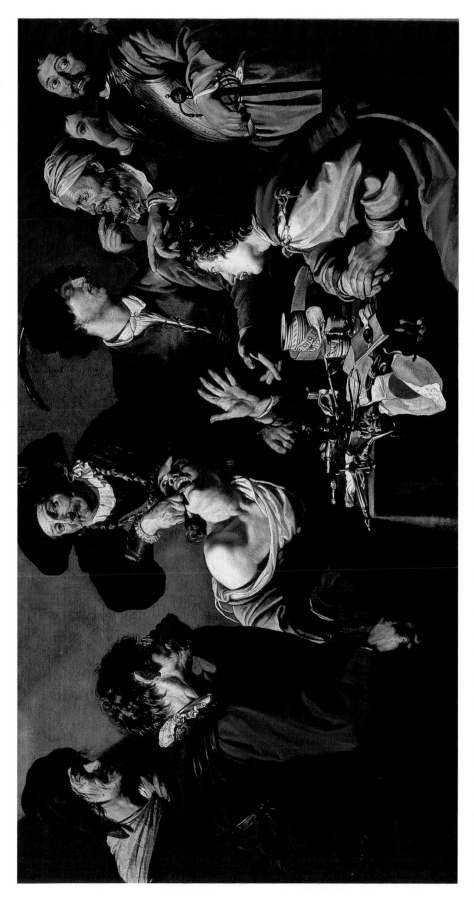

The Tooth Puller (early 17th century) by Theodor Rombouts. Oil on canvas, 116.2 cm × 221 cm. *Madrid, Museo Nacional del Prado.*

27

The Leech Woman *or* The Bloodletting (1660)
by Quirijn van Brekelenkam

Up to the 18th century, physicians and surgeons were limited to a few procedures for treating their patients, and these all had a long history. Apart from elective surgery, such as circumcision, cutting for the stone and trephination (for whatever cause), other procedures included cauterization, bloodletting, and the Chinese-derived techniques of moxibustion and acupuncture. Bloodletting was used for a variety of conditions in the belief that it released humours and toxins from the body. This could be achieved by phlebotomy, whereby a lancet or other means was used to incise a vein. Less dramatic techniques were the application of leeches, skin scarification or, as here, the application of a warmed cup to raise a blister. This is beautifully illustrated in this painting, the prominent candle being used to heat the cups, which are then applied to the young lady's arm.

The artist Quirijn van Brekelenkam (c 1620–c 1669) was a renowned Dutch painter, often of everyday scenes. He was always poor, and with a large family of nine children to support he acquired an additional job as a licensee to sell beer and brandy. He was very prolific, producing several hundred paintings in his short life. Unlike many other genre artists of the period, he conveyed the meaning of his work directly by the actual composition rather than through symbolic and literary references. In this painting there is not the ambiguity that is present in many other works of the period depicting a doctor visiting a patient.

The technique of bloodletting often did far more harm than good. In the case of George Washington, the elected first President of the United States, phlebotomy doubtless hastened his death in 1799. Thereafter the procedure was gradually abandoned by the profession.

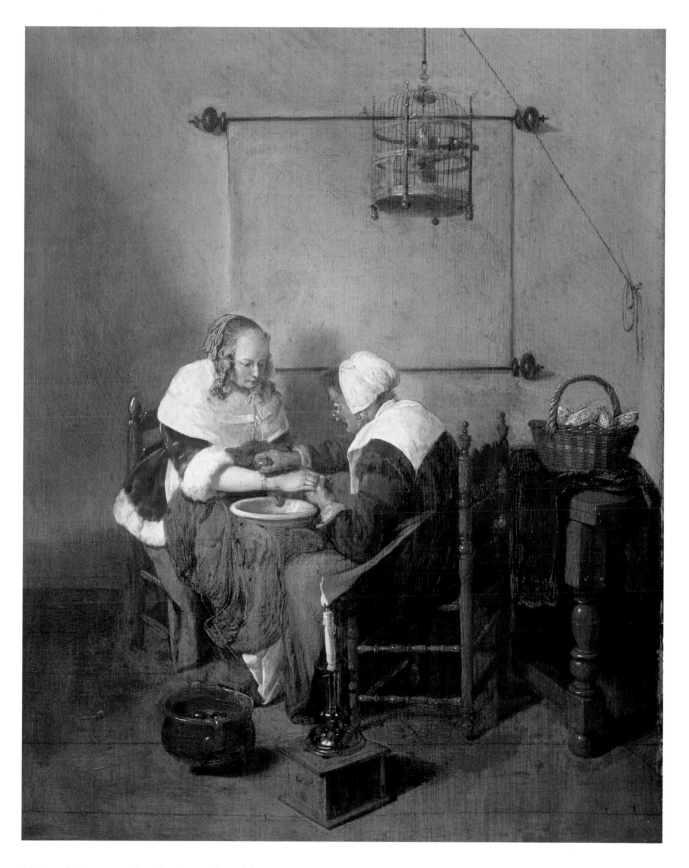

The Leech Woman or **The Bloodletting** (1660) by Quirijn van Brekelenkam. Oil on panel, 47.9 cm × 37 cm. *The Hague, Royal Cabinet of Paintings, Mauritshuis.*

28

The Wounded Man (c 1752)

by Gaspare Traversi

Gaspare Traversi was born in Naples around 1722 but spent much of his working life in Rome, where he died in 1770. He was influenced by a number of naturalist painters, such as Jusepe de Ribera, often remembered for his portrait of a begging street urchin with a club-foot. Traversi was also much influenced by Caravaggio, in whose work lighting was used with dramatic effect. Although he did paint a number of fine religious works, he is also noted for his scenes of everyday family life and customs. Here, for instance, a man has been wounded, the grief-stricken parents are just visible in the background and a weeping girl gently holds his head against her shoulder in order to comfort him. But especially interesting is the apparent professional detachment of the doctor, who very carefully and gently removes the overlying clothing in order to examine the wound more carefully. The assistant turns away as if realizing that any treatment will be useless. This must have so often been the case before the advent of appropriate surgical techniques and means of combating infection.

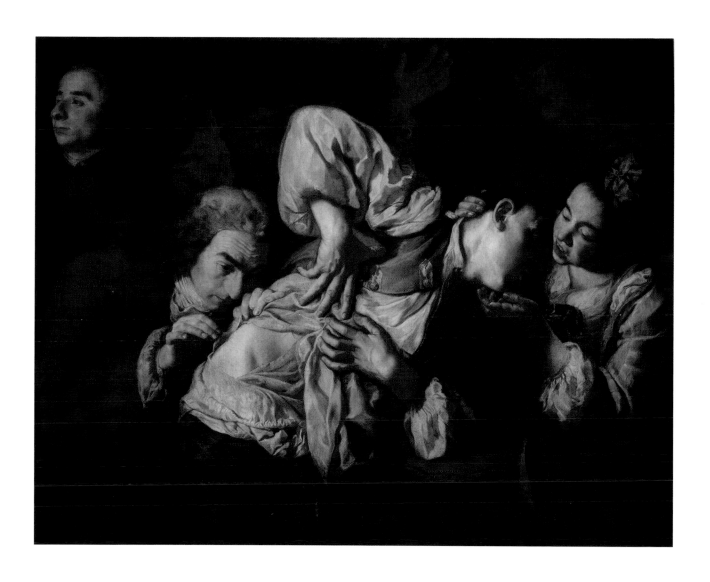

The Wounded Man (c 1752) by Gaspare Traversi. Oil on canvas, 101 cm × 127 cm. *Venice, Accademia.*
© 1990, Photo Scala, Florence, courtesy of the Ministero per i Beni e le Attività Culturali.

29

El Médico (The Doctor) (1779)

by Francisco José de Goya y Lucientes

Goya (1746–1828) was born in a small village near Saragossa. It was in Saragossa where he became an apprenticed artist and met the painter Francisco Bayeu, whose sister he later married. At the time, Bayeu was much respected for his work and became director of the tapestry workshops at the Royal Palace in Madrid, where Goya later joined him. This early work of Goya was in fact meant as a design for a tapestry and was executed under the direction of his brother-in-law, who instructed him in the necessary techniques as well as determining the subject and style of the work. The tapestry was planned to hang high over a door, which explains the low viewpoint and simple design and bold palette. Goya did several tapestry cartoons, but it seems that he did not find this sufficiently satisfying and later went on to pursue more imaginative and challenging projects.

This work shows a doctor, dressed in an appropriately coloured red cloak, seated and warming himself at a brazier. The open books imply his learning and his two apprentice (?) youths appear to be listening intently to him. In the early 19th century and even later, students of medicine were often apprenticed to a physician, as, for example, was Keats before he turned his attention more to poetry. Goya appears to have had a close relationship with the profession, as evidenced in his *Self-Portrait with Dr Arrieta,* painted many years later in 1820.

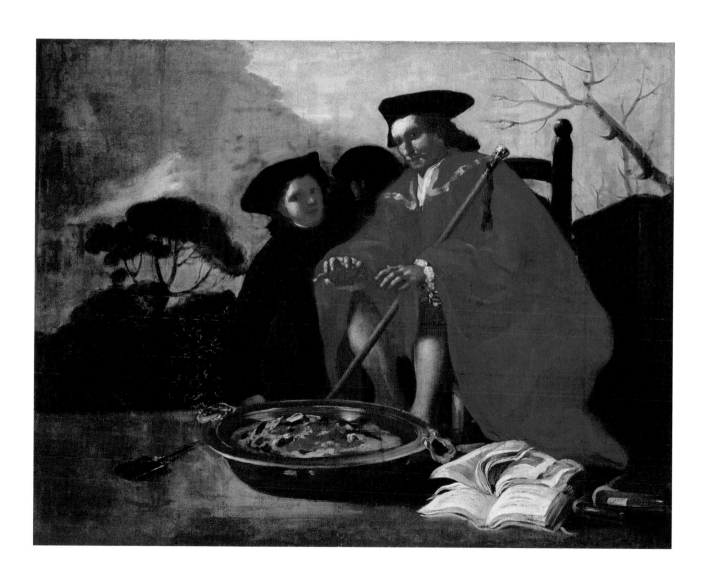

El Médico (The Doctor) (1779) by Francisco José de Goya y Lucientes. Oil on canvas, 95.8 cm × 120.2 cm. *Edinburgh, National Gallery of Scotland.*

30

The Cow Pock *or* The Wonderful Effects of the New Inoculation (1802)

by James Gillray

Smallpox was a global problem until 1979, by which time it had been totally eradicated by worldwide vaccination programmes. The story of the conferment of immunity to the disease can be traced back to ancient China and the practice of variolation, whereby a small amount of smallpox material from an infected person was scratched into the skin or blown up the nose. This technique was promoted in Britain in the 18th century by Lady Mary Wortley Montagu (1689–1762), who had been impressed by its effects during her travels in the Middle East. It was soon taken up with considerable enthusiasm by, for example, Robert Sutton (1707–1788) in England and Johnnie Williamson (1740–1803) in Shetland. But it was vaccination (from the Latin *vacca* for cow), introduced by Edward Jenner (1749–1823), that proved more agreeable and more effective. It had been known for many years that dairy-maids who had been infected with cowpox (a mild infection in humans) were immune to smallpox. The story is now well known of the West Country doctor Edward Jenner who, in May 1796, experimentally inoculated an eight-year-old local boy with cowpox material from an infected milkmaid and then later inoculated the boy with smallpox with no effect. Such an experiment nowadays would of course be fraught with serious ethical problems.

Jenner extended his studies to several other cases and published his results in 1798. The technique was soon extended to the populations of England and France and proved very effective in eradicating the disease. Napoleon in fact immunized his entire army. But that material from a cow, though indirectly, was being injected into humans was an abomination to some, including several church leaders. James Gillray (1757–1815) took the opportunity to lampoon the technique, as illustrated in this engraving. His name is often linked to other artists of around the time, such as Hogarth and subsequently George Cruikshank and Thomas Rowlandson, who in their work were especially critical of the profession, quackery and the gullibility of patients. Gillray was particularly noted for his cartoons of the Napoleonic Wars and, though scurrilous, his work was skilful.

In this work, he has depicted those being vaccinated with cowpox as then developing bovine features and even excreting and vomiting fully formed miniature cows! The lady to be vaccinated is clearly apprehensive. But, despite its critics, the practice soon gained acceptance and spread widely throughout the world, leading eventually to the total eradication of the disease and a model for what may be achieved by international cooperation.

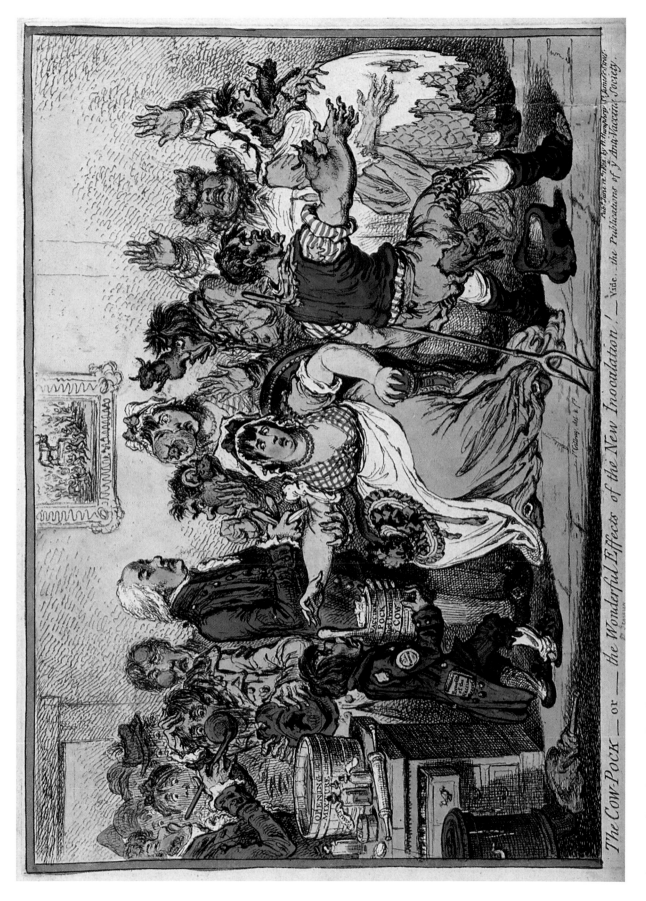

The Cow Pock or The Wonderful Effects of the New Inoculation (1802) by James Gillray. Etching with water-colour, 24.8 cm × 34.9 cm London, Wellcome Library.

31

The Mummy State (c 1822–1841)

anonymous

It has been said that pneumonia is probably one of the very earliest serious diseases to have afflicted humans. Pneumococcal organisms have been found in prehistoric remains and evidence of the disease has been observed in Egyptian mummies from 1200 BC. Its effects were particularly devastating in the very young and the elderly, and by the beginning of the last century William Osler noted that the death rate, in those over 60, was around 70%. He commented '...one may say that to die of pneumonia is almost the natural end of old people' – often a painless end, which Osler himself referred to as 'the friend of the aged'.

René Laënnec's introduction of the stethoscope in 1816 was a major step forward in diagnosing pulmonary diseases, later aided by X-radiography (discovered by Wilhelm Roentgen in 1895), and the first of the causative agents, the pneumococcus, was identified in the early 1880s. But not until the advent of sulphonamides, and later penicillin in the 1940s, was there an effective cure. Up until then, a common approach was to 'sweat it out' of the patient by keeping him warm with blankets, hot-water bottles and so on, and he was forced to drink plenty of fluids. This is satirized in this coloured etching of around 1822–1841. The lettering accompanying the work states 'The patient ... is tightly enveloped in blankets to perspire if he lives long enough. He is usually made a Mummy of or cured, the chances are equal'.

Without a specific treatment, pyrexia persisted until around 7–10 days, when a 'crisis' occurred and the patient either died or his temperature fell and he recovered. The physician, relatives and even the patient were often well aware of this course and awaited the crisis with considerable trepidation. Fortunately, with modern treatments this is often now a thing of the past, although in those who are immunologically compromised in any way, the mortality rate is still significant.

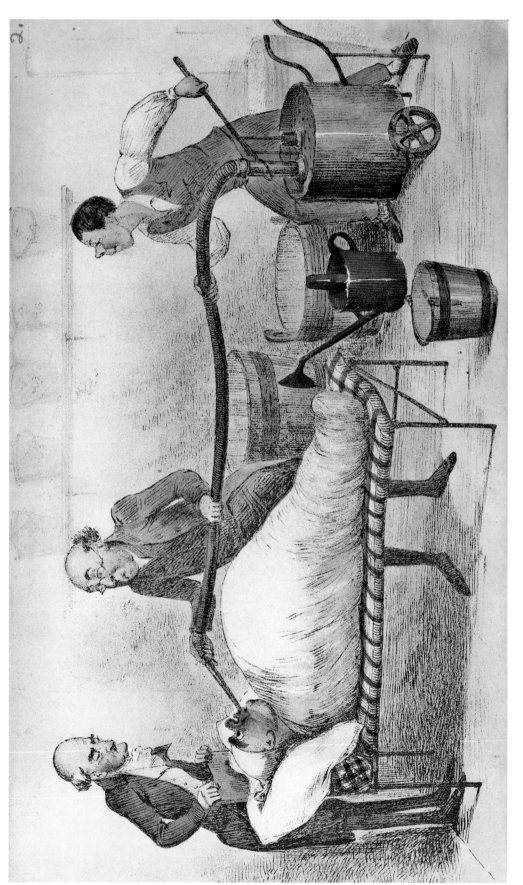

The Mummy State (c 1822–1841), anonymous. Hand-coloured etching, 12.1 cm × 21 cm. *London, Museum of the Royal Pharmaceutical Society of Great Britain.*

32

Robert Macaire Mesmerises an Old Lady in Front of an Audience (1829–1841)

by Honoré Daumier

Franz Anton Mesmer (1734–1815), who gave his name to mesmerism or animal magnetism, later called hypnotism, had a very chequered career. He studied medicine in Vienna and his doctoral thesis was on the medical effects of the influence of the planets. He later developed a novel and unorthodox healing practice that depended on placing magnets over critical parts of the body. His methods were considered unprofessional and he left for Paris, where he developed fashionable séances for nervous women using his animal magnetism, during which some would become 'mesmerized' into a hypnotic trance. He claimed that his techniques and methods cured all manner of conditions, including paralysis, gout and accidental deafness. But Mesmer was also seen in France as a quack and was obliged to leave. At first his ideas did a little better in London, but eventually here too he became discredited, and he died in obscurity. Mozart, in 1790, actually had a character in his opera *Cosi fan Tutti* disguise herself as a Dr Mesmer.

Honoré Daumier (1808–1879) was a renowned French satirist. In his many lithographs and drawings a Dr Robert Macaire often featured. This was a fictional character of ridicule in a melodrama running in Paris at the time and was often used by Daumier in deriding unprofessional doctors, dentists and surgeons, and unscrupulous lawyers and bankers. His work did not sell well and he remained poor throughout his life. In old age he became blind as a result of a failed cataract operation. Monet subsequently fared much better when he underwent such an operation several years later.

In 1843, some years after Mesmer's death, James Braid, a Manchester surgeon, coined the word *hypnotism* for 'animal magnetism', a term that has persisted ever since. The technique was once indicated as a method to induce relaxation, or to relieve symptoms of hysteria or even as an aid to psychotherapy. But none of these approaches has proved helpful in the long term, and they are no longer recommended in present-day clinical psychiatry.

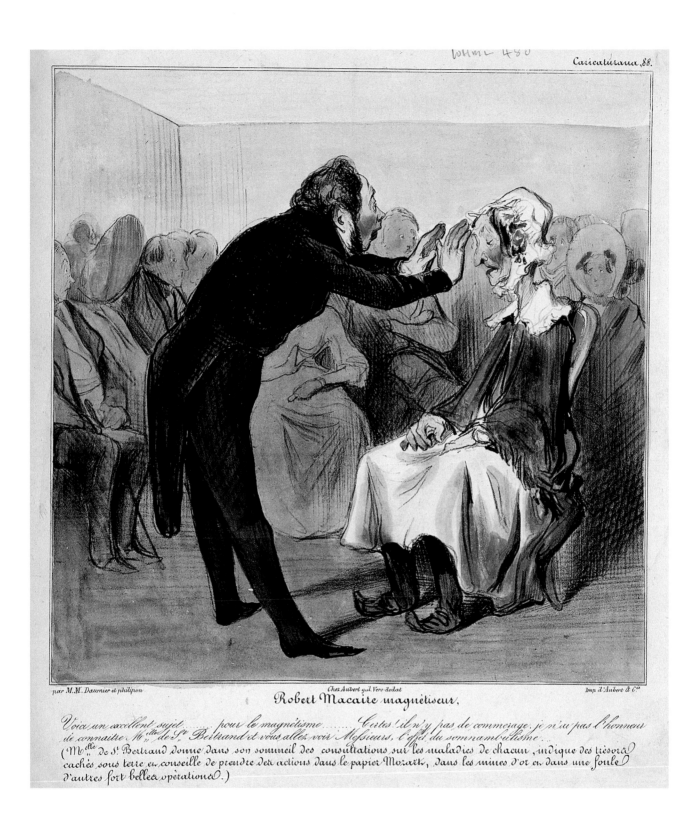

Robert Macaire Mesmerises an Old Lady in Front of an Audience (1829–1841) by Honoré Daumier. Coloured lithograph, 23.6 cm × 23.1 cm. *London, Wellcome Library.*

33

The Phrenologist (1825)
by 'E. H.' (? Edward Hull)

Edward Hull was a lithographer who flourished in London from 1820 to 1834, but little else is known of him. However, the Wellcome Library in London has several other prints of his that also relate to medical matters. The main interest here, however, is the topic that he is illustrating, namely phrenology, whereby it was thought that various brain functions (mental and moral) could be related to parts of the overlying skull. The concept had been introduced by Franz Joseph Gall (1758–1828). He was born in Germany and completed his medical studies in Vienna, where he became a well-established physician. He began to propagate his theory of the relationship of bumps on the skull to different cerebral functions in 1792, eventually defining no less than 27 faculties in this way, and went on to elaborate the theory to explain differences between animal and human brains. He subsequently published a massive four-volume work on the subject, copiously illustrated with detailed copperplate engravings.

Gall's theory was based on studies of the cranial features of people from the extremes of society: from great writers, poets, musicians and mathematicians to lunatics, criminals and the deaf and blind. In all of his work he was assisted by Johann Spurzheim, who went on to develop his own phrenological system.

But by the early 19th century, phrenology was on the wane. The main attack came from those who pointed out that brain injuries rarely affect faculties in a way predicted by phrenology. Similar conclusions were drawn from experimental animal studies. Thus, by the time this lithograph was produced, phrenology was seen as quackery and satirized in many contemporary works throughout Europe and North America, most notably in Britain by Thomas Rowlandson. In this lithograph Gall is seen examining the head of a pretty girl. The men waiting in line are grotesquely portrayed, as is Gall himself. But it was Paul Broca (1824–1880) of Paris who was one of the first to apply a rational approach to the subject. In 1861, he drew attention to the speech centre after studying the case of a man with uncontrollable epilepsy and a serious speech defect. At autopsy, the man was shown to have a 'chronic progressive softening' of the third frontal convolution of the left hemisphere, later known as Broca's area. This localization was subsequently confirmed by Hughlings Jackson. Later, further areas of cerebral localization emerged from studying patients with specific defects as a result of disease or trauma, thus opening up the development of neurology and particularly neurosurgery. Nevertheless, despite the preposterous claims of the phrenologists, at least Gall had contributed to the detachment of mental function from philosophy and in this regard, deserves credit.

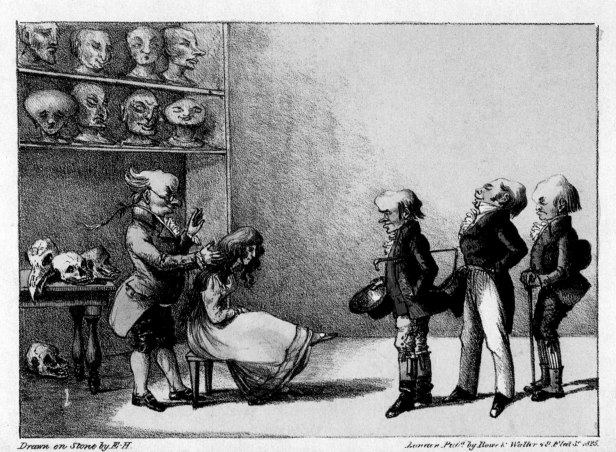

Drawn on Stone by E.H.

London Pub.d by Rowe & Walter 49 Fleet St 1825.

THE PHRENOLOGIST.

The Phrenologist (1825) by 'E. H.' (? Edward Hull). Coloured lithograph, 13.2 cm × 18.4 cm. *London, Wellcome Library.*

34

Portrait of Sir Alexander Morison (1852)
by Richard Dadd

Both the subject of this painting and the artist himself are of medical interest. Richard Dadd (1817–1886) was an English painter who in his early career produced some notable work when, in 1842, he accompanied Sir Thomas Phillips as a travelling companion on a Grand Tour of Europe and the Middle East. However, towards the end of the tour, Dadd began to develop alarmingly aggressive behaviour and suffered delusions of persecution. On returning to Britain, he had an unprovoked argument with his father, whom he viciously attacked and killed. He then escaped to France, only to attempt to kill a complete stranger. He was arrested and extradited to England, where he was found to be unfit to plead because of insanity. This was around the time (1843) that the McNaghten rules were introduced whereby a convicted murderer could escape capital punishment if it could be proved that he was insane at the time of the crime. This was certainly true in the case of Richard Dadd, and in 1844 he was committed first to the Criminal Lunatic Asylum at Bethlem Hospital and later to Broadmoor Hospital, where he spent the rest of his life. He continued to be deluded and deranged, and may well have suffered from schizophrenia, a disorder that is likely to have also affected a brother and sister. However, he was encouraged to resume his painting by, among others, Dr Alexander Morison, a Scottish physician who was then at the Bethlem Hospital. There is little doubt that encouraging Dadd to paint had a beneficial calming effect. This more humane approach reflected the change in attitude to the care of the insane at the time.

Dr (later Sir) Alexander Morison was one of the first physicians in Britain to become involved in the care of the mentally ill in the newly created asylums. These Medical Superintendents or 'mental alienists' were the forerunners of the specialty of psychiatry. In 1840, Morison authored one of the very first textbooks on mental illness, which was still related by many physicians to physiognomy and phrenology. It is a beautifully illustrated book with crayon drawings and watercolours of his patients that clearly depict, among other disorders, cases of microcephaly. The fascinating relationship between Dadd and Morison was the subject of an exhibition at the Scottish National Portrait Gallery in 1980. In this painting the doctor is placed against a background of, probably, Newhaven by Edinburgh, with the inclusion of two fishwives – a background that may have been suggested by Morison himself or from a contemporary illustration.

Although he continued to paint in Broadmoor throughout his life, Dadd's work remained original and un-influenced by the current movements of the Pre-Raphaelites in Britain or the Impressionists in France. Many of his works nowadays occupy prominent positions in several galleries, including the Tate Britain, the Victoria and Albert Museum, the British Museum and the Ashmolean Museum, Oxford.

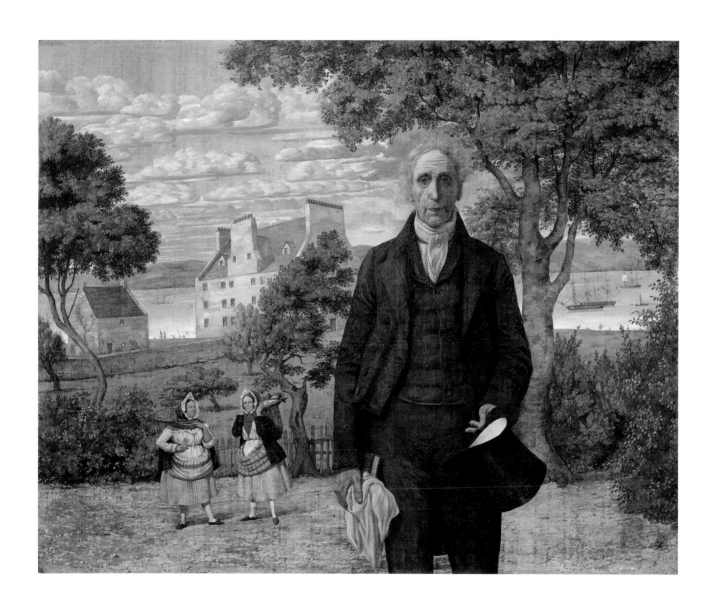

Portrait of Sir Alexander Morison (1852) by Richard Dadd. Oil on canvas, 51.1 cm × 61.3 cm. *Edinburgh, Scottish National Portrait Gallery.*

35

The Death of Chatterton (1856)

by Henry Wallis

This tragic scene, epitomizing a young poet dying alone in a garret, seems a peculiar choice for a series concerned with medical treatment. But appearances can be misleading.

Thomas Chatterton (1752–1770) was the posthumous child of an impoverished Bristol schoolmaster. He was somewhat backward as a child, only learning to read when he was eight. Soon afterwards, however, he began to write strange poems. He gained access to a room of deeds in the Church of St Mary Redcliffe, where he familiarized himself with the old style of handwriting and archaic spelling. Subsequently, he began to fabricate poems which he attributed to a Thomas Rowley, a 15th century priest, as well as other notables. But he was unsuccessful in convincing publishers and lived cold, hungry and in great poverty in a Holborn garret. On 24 August 1770, just three months short of 18, he took poison and was found dead by his landlady surrounded by torn manuscripts. He was interred as a pauper in the workhouse cemetery in Shoe Lane.

It was generally assumed that he had taken his own life by swallowing arsenic, which was identified as the cause of death at the time. However, more recent commentators have suggested that it was the result of a failed attempt to cure syphilis. Certainly he was sexually precocious and had a number of liaisons with girls in Bristol and later in London. At the time, only crude preparations of mercury or even arsenic were considered treatments for syphilis, neither being effective. It was often said that one night with Venus meant months with Mercury. It was not until the advent of salvarsan (Ehrlich's compound 606) in the early 1900s, and particularly penicillin in the 1940s, that truly effective treatment became possible.

Incidentally, George Meredith (1828–1909), an acquaintance of Henry Wallis, posed for the painting, there being no surviving portrait of Chatterton. Meredith himself was a poet and novelist, and the picture was actually painted in Chatterton's garret. Henry Wallis (1830–1916) was a minor English pre-Raphaelite painter and his Chatterton painting won him enormous popularity at the time. Two years after completing this work, he eloped to Capri with Meredith's wife.

Whatever the tragic circumstances surrounding this painting, the image remains that of a gifted penniless youth dying alone and unrecognized: a romantic icon for someone totally dedicated to his or her art.

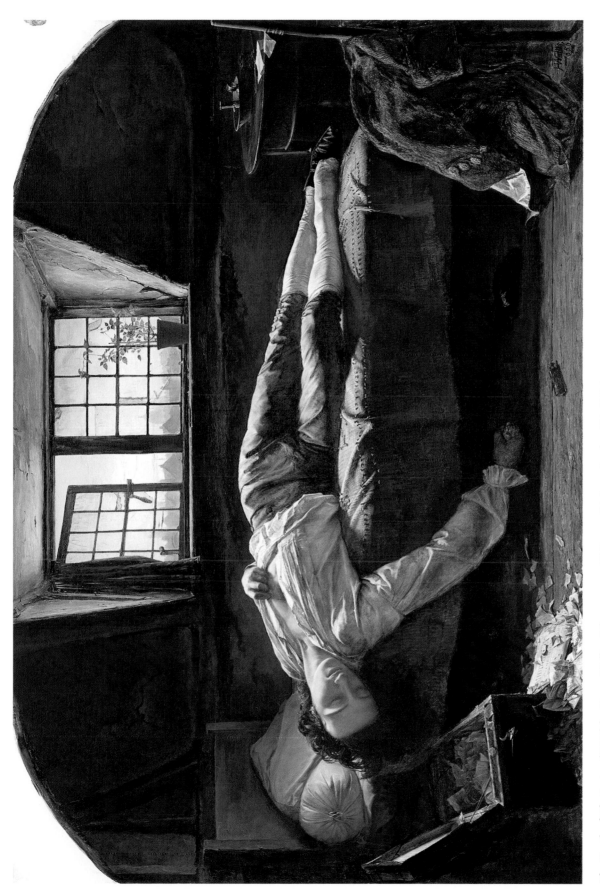

The Death of Chatterton (1856) by Henry Wallis. Oil on canvas, 62.7 cm × 94.1 cm. *London, Tate Britain.*
© Tate, London 2005.

36

Amputation (1793)

by Thomas Rowlandson

Thomas Rowlandson (1756–1827) is now renowned for his etchings and watercolours so very critical of the profession, quackery and the innocent gullibility of patients in 18th century Britain. He produced more than one hundred such works. He would certainly have antagonized many professionals; nevertheless, he did have many medical friends and a frequent supper companion was a Dr John Wolcot, who probably provided him with many first-hand ideas for his work.

Amputation, before the era of anaesthetics, was a terrifying experience for the patient and a daunting and demanding ordeal for the surgeon. The aim was to conclude the surgery as quickly as possible, which required considerable skill and manual dexterity. One renowned Scottish surgeon of the time is said to have completed the procedure in less than a minute, but in the course of it he removed the thumb of an assistant! Haemorrhage was controlled by a tourniquet (but apparently not in this illustration). The post-operative mortality approached 50% due to blood loss and infection. St Anthony's fire (erysipelas) occurred almost invariably after surgery right up until the late 19th century. In a graphic coloured woodcut of 1517 by Johann Wechtlin of an amputation, a bystander has a moistened animal bladder over an amputation stump with a Greek letter *tau* to indicate he suffers from St Anthony's fire, one form of post-surgical infection. Others included gangrene, septicaemia and pyaemia.

In this work, skeletons litter the surgery, making it redolent of a dissecting room. On the wall is a list of approved surgeons, including Sir Valiant Venery, Dr Peter Putrid, Launcelot Slashmuscle and Benjamin Boweles. The surgeon wears a carpenter's apron and is made to seem as if he is sawing a piece of wood. The assistant on the left holds a crutch for the patient's subsequent use.

But whatever the apparent barbarity of surgical amputation, at the time before the era of anaesthetics and antisepsis, the surgeon was left with little alternative when faced with a life-threatening diseased member.

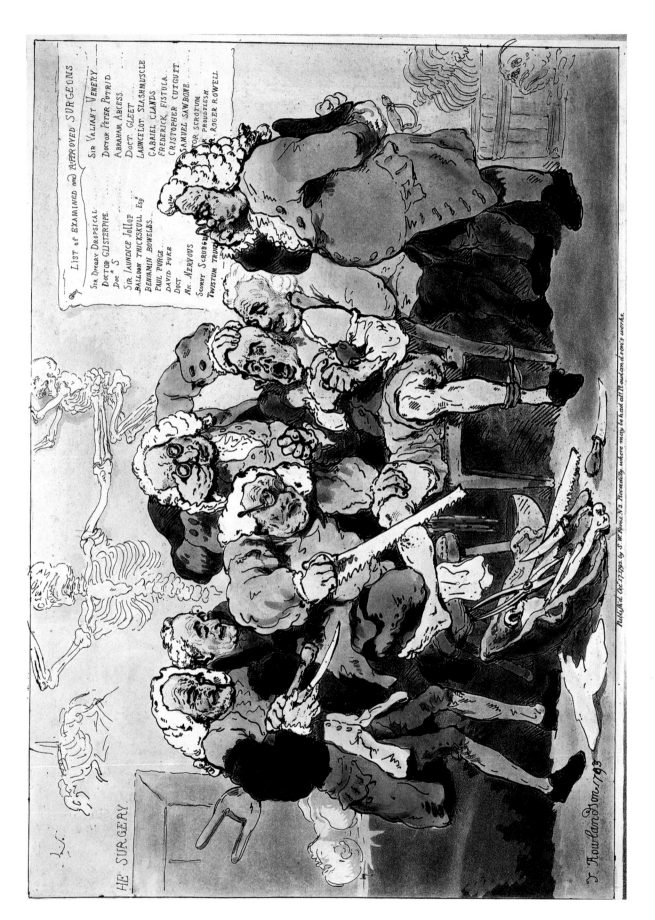

Amputation (1793) by Thomas Rowlandson. Etching with watercolour, 27.8 cm × 40.3 cm. *London, Wellcome Library.*

37

First Successful Public Demonstration of Surgical Anaesthesia (1882)

by Robert C. Hinckley

Methods for the alleviation of pain, from whatever cause, go back a long way and have involved a variety of techniques, including incantations and similar devices. But certainly in the case of surgical operations, reliance was placed on the value of various herbal preparations, such as opium, cannabis, mandrake and henbane. Alcohol played a large part, the patient often being totally intoxicated by the time an amputation, for example, was attempted.

What proved to be the most important development, namely inhalation anaesthesia, can be dated from the late 1790s with Humphry Davy's finding of the painkilling properties of nitrous oxide inhalation. But it was the subsequent revelation that ether had similar properties that really paved the way for effective anaesthesia. Credit is usually given to W. T. G. Morton in this regard, although others have also been cited. The method was convincingly used for the first time in general surgery on 16 October 1846, at the Massachusetts General Hospital. Some would argue that this is the most memorable date in the history of surgery. Robert C. Hinckley (1853–1941), a prominent American portrait painter of the time, completed this work some years after the actual event. Here, we see the 68-year-old celebrated surgeon John Collins Warren, Professor of Surgery at Harvard Medical School, removing a tumour from the jaw of a young Gilbert Abbot. Morton himself stands behind the patient administering ether through a specially designed glass apparatus. The operation was completed painlessly in 25 minutes to Warren's celebrated exclamation, 'Gentlemen, this is no humbug'. News travelled quickly and Liston in London used ether anaesthesia for a leg amputation in December of the same year.

However, the following year, James Young Simpson (1811–1870), Professor of Midwifery in Edinburgh, showed that chloroform was a more effective and preferred agent and was used for the first time with great success by him in November 1847.

Meanwhile, John Snow (1813–1858), celebrated for the curtailment of an outbreak of cholera in London in 1854 by removing the handle of the water pump in Broad Street, Soho, was also an accomplished anaesthetist in operations from simple tooth extractions to major operations, such as mastectomy. It has been estimated that he anaesthetized over 5000 cases in a dozen years and became particularly famous for his use of chloroform in obstetrics. In fact, he gave chloroform successfully to Queen Victoria at the birth of her son Leopold, which popularized the technique throughout Britain and Europe. When he succumbed to a stroke in June 1858, Snow was characteristically working on his maqnum opus *On Chloroform*. Incidentally, he frequently employed intubation during anaesthesia.

Of course, the story didn't end there, for many major advances have occurred since, with the introduction of other agents, including halothane and its derivatives. Concomitantly, various intravenous anaesthetic agents have been developed to be used alone or more commonly for induction of general anaesthesia.

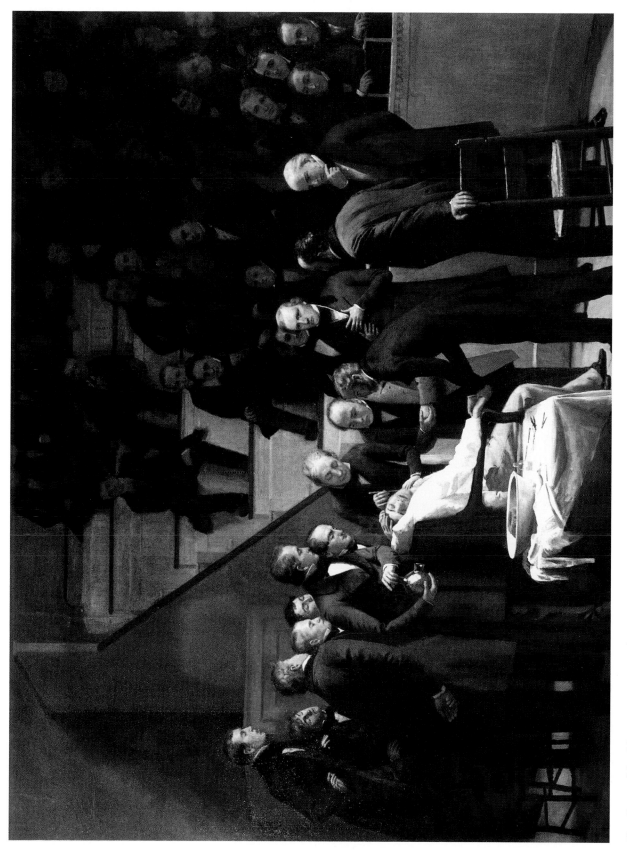

First Successful Public Demonstration of Surgical Anaesthesia (1882) by Robert C. Hinckley. Oil on canvas, 243.8 cm × 292.1 cm. *Massachusetts, Boston Medical Library in the Francis A. Countway Library of Medicine.*

38

First Use of Ether Anaesthesia in Britain, 1846 (nd)

anonymous

This photograph is of a work by an unknown artist. It was commissioned by Sir Henry Wellcome (1853–1936) and hung in University College Hospital. The painting, however, no longer exists – only a poor black-and-white photograph of the work has been found on a wall at the hospital. On the reverse of this is written a note stating that the Trustees of Sir Henry Wellcome had had the actual painting destroyed because it contained some inaccuracies, but nothing to indicate what these inaccuracies were or when it was destroyed.

In the scene, the eminent surgeon Robert Liston (1794–1847) is operating. He studied medicine at Edinburgh University and was a friend and colleague of James Syme, both eventually becoming distinguished surgeons. Except for a very brief period, Syme remained in Edinburgh but Liston left for London in 1835 to become Professor of Clinical Surgery and was elected a Fellow of the Royal Society in 1841. He quickly developed a reputation for his dexterity and resourcefulness. In this painting, Liston stands ready with his knife to perform an amputation for osteomyelitis on a 36-year-old butler, Frederick Churchill. The operation took place on 21 December 1846 and was the first use of anaesthesia in Britain. William Squire, a 21-year-old medical student, administers the anaesthetic to the patient from an apparatus made for the purpose by his uncle Peter Squire, a local pharmacist. A young Joseph Lister, then studying for a BA degree and merely a spectator of the event who would not qualify in medicine until 1852, stands at the left of the painting and is seen in profile facing Liston. The actual amputation took less than a minute to perform and the whole procedure was completed in less than five minutes, the patient being completely unaware of what had happened. Liston, clearly excited and delighted, exclaimed, 'This Yankee dodge, gentlemen, beats mesmerism hollow'!

This is a fascinating painting that commemorates one of the greatest and most important achievements in British surgery.

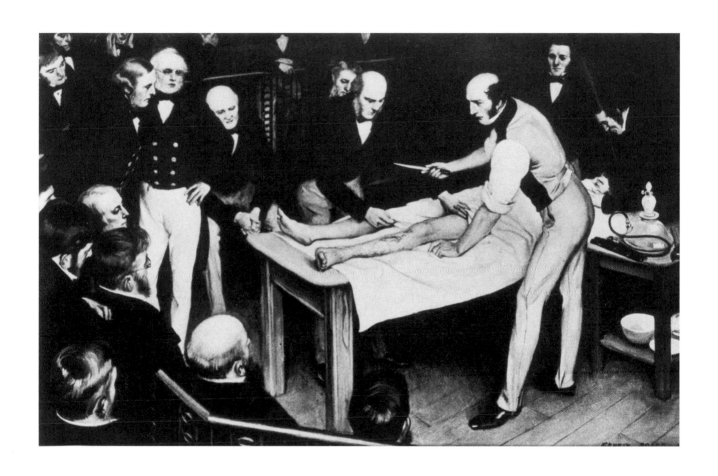

The First Use of Ether Anaesthesia in Britain, 1846 (nd), anonymous. *London, UCL Art Collections, University College London.*

39

The Gross Clinic (1875)

by Thomas Eakins

The great American painter Thomas Eakins (1844–1916) studied at the Pennsylvania Academy of the Fine Arts and then in Paris at the École des Beaux-Arts and later Spain, finally settling in Philadelphia in 1870. He made his career in painting portraits of those he chose and represented his subjects in powerful but often unflattering physical and psychological terms.

In 1875, inspired by the approaching Centennial celebrations and exhibition of national subjects, Eakins painted *The Gross Clinic*. Here, he portrayed the internationally celebrated Philadelphia surgeon Professor Samuel Gross in an operation for osteomyelitis at Jefferson Medical College. To the left of the surgeon, Dr West, the clerk, takes notes impassively. Below and to the left, a woman (perhaps the patient's mother) is seen cringing and covering her eyes from the horrifying scene. In those days, close relatives could be present when charity patients were operated on. Although this was intended as a tribute to advances in American surgery, the jury rejected the work. It was seen as being too distressing and unpleasant.

Eakins, however, did reveal a great deal about surgery at the time. General anaesthesia was now given and the anaesthetist at the head of the table administers open-drop anaesthesia (the Schimmelbusch mask was introduced a little later). The surgeon and his staff wear ordinary everyday frock-coats, and there is nowhere any evidence of sterility, and the equipment lies on an exposed table in the foreground. Yet Lister had introduced antiseptic procedures some eight years previously. Samuel Gross, like many other surgeons at the time, refused to accept the evidence of infection. Perhaps the concepts of the germ theory were seen as too 'scientific' and the demanding and painstaking antiseptic method of surgery, unacceptable. It would be many years before the theory was widely accepted in American surgery. But whatever the academic merits of the work, *The Gross Clinic* remains a very fine portrait of an outstanding surgeon.

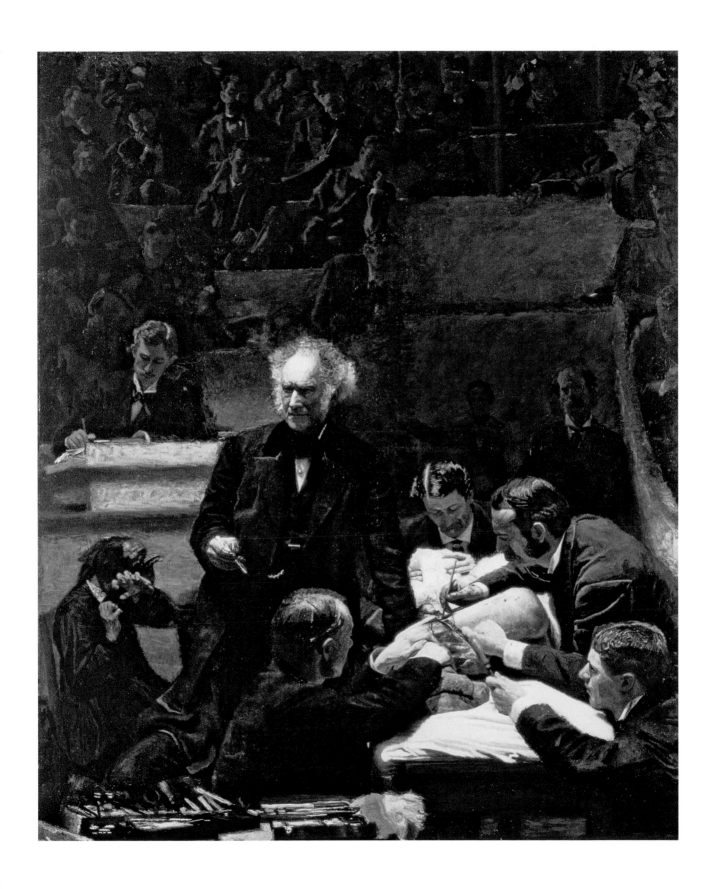

The Gross Clinic (1875) by Thomas Eakins. Oil on canvas, 243.8 cm × 198.1 cm. *Philadelphia, Thomas Jefferson University.*

40

The Improvised Field Hospital (1865)
by Jean-Frédéric Bazille

This work is interesting not only from a medical point of view but also because both the painter and his subject were artists who trained together under Charles Gleyre in Paris, and in fact at one time shared a studio. The subject was Claude Monet (1840–1926), particularly famous for his paintings of the water lilies in his garden at Giverny, who had had an accidental injury in Chailly near Fontainebleau in 1865. This prevented him from painting and he became confined to bed. At the time, he was chronically short of money and relied heavily for financial help and support from his close friend Jean-Frédéric Bazille (1841–1870), who came from a prosperous old bourgeois family from Montpellier in the South of France. After beginning a medical career in Paris, Bazille studied painting and became a close friend of many of the well-known painters of the time, including Manet, Renoir and Sisley. He showed great talent as an artist, as illustrated in this painting, and gave up medicine in 1865, but his promising career was cut short at the age of 29 when he was killed by a stray bullet during the Franco-Prussian War.

From the painting, it seems that Monet has cellulitis of the lower leg, and since this was well before the era of antibiotics, treatment for such an infection was often palliative. It seems that perhaps the earthenware jar is suspended in such a way as to allow its contents to drip onto the affected wound. Although this is pure speculation, could this have been an arrangement for a drip of carbolic acid (phenol) for its antiseptic properties? James Lister's first trial of carbolic acid treatment for an infected wound was in August 1865 and he subsequently reported several successfully treated cases in his celebrated *Lancet* article in 1867. However, this was France and a Frenchman, François-Jules Lemaire (1814–1886) had already recommended this approach to the treatment of infected wounds in 1860, about the same time as did Frank Calvert, Professor of Chemistry in Manchester. So it is possible that this is what we are seeing in this picture. Incidentally, Lister seems to have been unaware of Lemaire's earlier work with carbolic acid. Whatever the case may be, clearly Monet overcame the infection, for he recovered completely and entered the most productive period of his entire life.

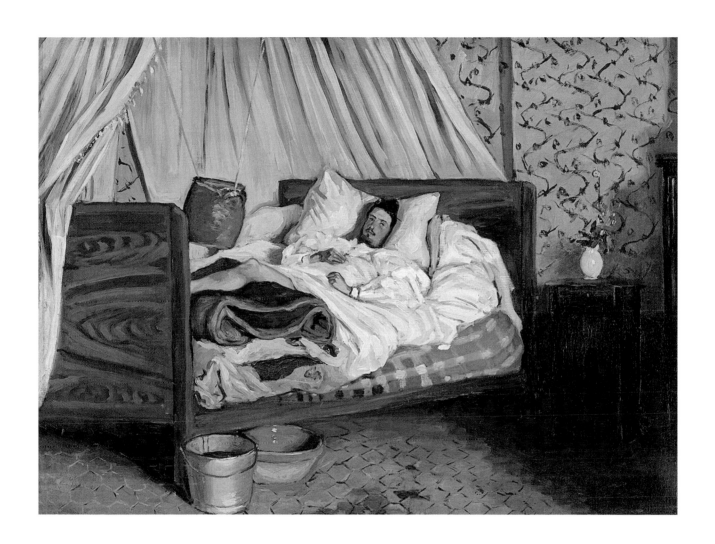

The Improvised Field Hospital (1865) by Jean-Frédéric Bazille. Oil on canvas, 47 cm × 65 cm. *Paris, Musée d'Orsay.*
© Photo RMN, © Hervé Lewandowski.

41

Antiseptic Surgery (1882)

by T. P. Collings

After the introduction of general anaesthesia in 1846, the next memorable date in the history of surgery is March 1865. Then, Joseph (later Lord) Lister (1827–1912), a prominent London-trained surgeon, accepting the implications of Louis Pasteur's (1822–1895) fermentation experiments, came to believe that bacteria could enter wounds from the environment. He therefore introduced his antiseptic system of surgery, using carbolic acid for the first time in the case of a severe compound fracture. He saved the limb, which otherwise would have been amputated. Two years later he published his classic paper 'On a new method of treating compound fractures' (*Lancet* 1867; **i**: 326–9), in which he described eleven amputation cases, in nine of which the limb was saved. For centuries, with only a few notable exceptions, such as Theodoric and Ambroise Paré, most surgeons believed that 'laudable pus' in wounds was to be encouraged. These days were now at an end.

Lister developed an array of antiseptic techniques involving apparatus for spraying carbolic acid onto the wound and surroundings during an operation, and subsequently using dressings soaked in the material. This is clearly illustrated in this wood engraving from William Watson Cheyne's text on antiseptic surgery published in 1882. Cheyne was the son of a sea captain and was born in Tasmania in 1852. He was brought to Scotland by his grandfather, who was a minister in Shetland. He studied medicine in Edinburgh, then became Lister's house surgeon and subsequently a pioneer of antiseptic surgery in Britain. In 1912, he became President of the Royal College of Surgeons. In this woodcut, it is clear that the entire environment of the operation is in a cloud of antiseptic spray. However, the surgeon and his assistants are still wearing their every-day clothing and do not wear gowns or surgical gloves. This will change over the next few years with the introduction of *aseptic* surgery.

Lister retired from the Chair of Clinical Surgery at King's College London at age 65 in 1892. In that year he and Pasteur met at the Sorbonne on the memorable occasion of the latter's 70th birthday on 27 December, when Lister paid a feeling tribute to the man to whose work he and surgery in general owed so much.

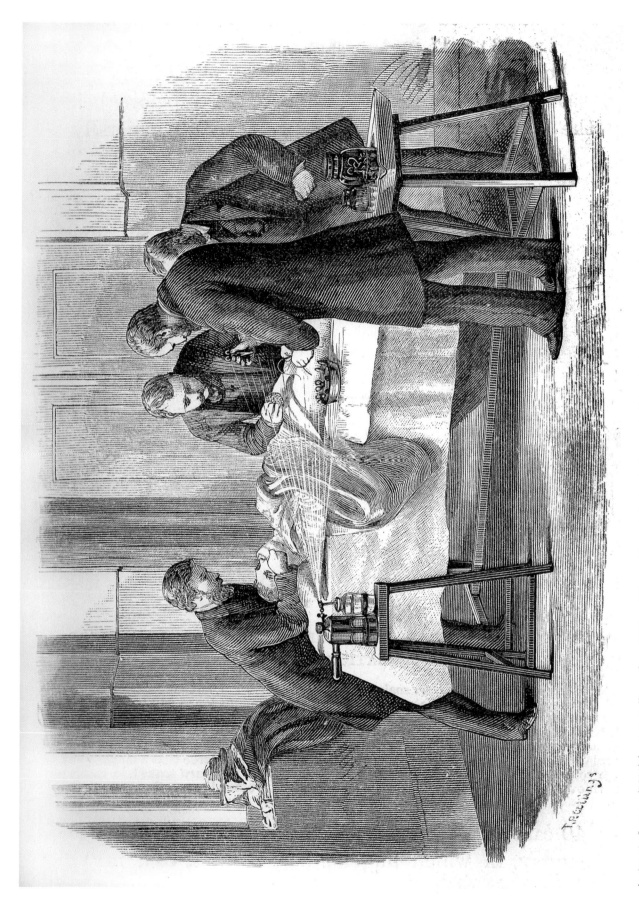

Antiseptic Surgery (1882) by T. P. Collings, from William Watson Cheyne's *Antiseptic Surgery: Its Principles, Practice, History and Results.* London: Smith, Elder, 1882: 71. Wood engraving, 11 cm × 13.5 cm. *London, Royal Society of Medicine Library.*

42

The Agnew Clinic (1889)

by Thomas Eakins

Lister's contribution to antiseptic surgery was immense, and although it was slow to be accepted by some, an enthusiastic following of surgeons developed, including Péan and Championnière in France, Saxtorph in Denmark, and several in Germany, among them Thiersch, Volkmann, Nussbaum, Billroth and Ernst von Bergmann, who was the first to introduce the term *asepsis*. Thus was ushered in the era of steam sterilization of instruments together with the wearing of gowns and masks. Surgical gloves were introduced in 1889 by the Johns Hopkins surgeon William Halstead, initially for his theatre sister (who later became his wife) because her hands were very sensitive to the antiseptic chemicals being used at the time.

In this painting, the surgeon and his assistants are operating on a woman's breast and are wearing white coats but not masks and apparently no surgical gloves, but clearly an effort is being made to maintain a degree of sterility. It depicts one of the most esteemed surgeons in 19th century America, D. Hayes Agnew, who taught at the University of Pennsylvania Medical School. On Agnew's retirement in 1889, his students commissioned a portrait to show the surgeon operating. As in the case of Eakins' earlier painting, *The Gross Clinic* (Plate 39), this work was also criticized at the time for being too realistic and unpleasant. But Eakins was more in sympathy with scientific ideas of the day than with aesthetic considerations. On one occasion the artist is reported to have forced some of his female students to face a nude as part of their training. He was severely criticized and discharged from the Academy and avoided by polite society. He sold practically no paintings during his lifetime. Now, however, we appreciate the merits of this great painting, reflecting as it does a surgeon involved in his craft toward the end of the 19th century. As the American poet Walt Whitman commented at the time, 'People who like Eakins best are people who have no art prejudices to interpose'.

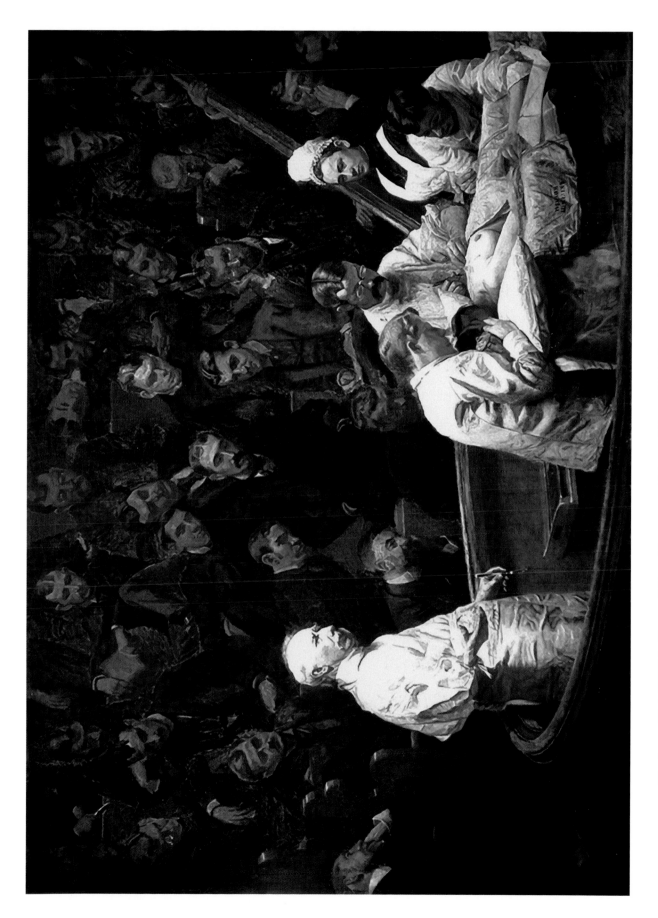

The Agnew Clinic (1889) by Thomas Eakins. Oil on canvas, 228 cm × 320 cm. *Philadelphia, University of Pennsylvania Art Collection.*

43

Theodor Billroth Operating (1890)
by Adalbert Franz Seligmann

By the latter part of the 19th century, German-speaking universities were internationally renowned for their advances in laboratory science, clinics and surgery. One of these centres was the Allgemeines Krankenhaus of the University of Vienna. Among its leaders was Theodor Billroth (1829–1894), one of the greatest surgeons of all time. In January 1881, he was the first to perform a successful gastrectomy with the patient surviving. He also pioneered the excision of tumours of the bladder and bowel and performed the first laryngectomy. Interestingly, he considered that cardiac surgery was never going to be a reality! He was also one of the very first to keep careful records of both his successes and failures. Study reveals that most of the 700 or so patients treated each year may have suffered from infections, frequently tuberculosis and syphilis, and various tumours or injuries. The overall mortality rate was around 10%, but it was considerably higher in the case of malignant tumours, although Billroth tended to favour a conservative approach in many such serious cases.

In this painting, Billroth is seen at the height of his fame when he was around 60 years of age. The patient's head is shaved, as the operation was a neurotomy for trigeminal neuralgia. The anaesthetic is being administered by an open-drop method, with a mixture of alcohol, chloroform and ether, favoured by Billroth. Although he was clearly attracted to the need for antisepsis, the surgeons do not wear masks or gloves. He was renowned for often entering the operating room with a large Havana cigar in his mouth, which he sometimes continued to smoke during the operation. This is a faithful depiction of surgery at the time by the artist Adalbert Franz Seligmann (1862–1945), a contemporary Viennese artist and friend.

Apart from surgery, Billroth was a very cultured man. He had hoped to pursue a career in music, but was dissuaded by his mother. Nevertheless, he continued to play the piano throughout his life and befriended many writers and musicians. Brahms was a particularly close friend of the surgeon, to whom he dedicated two of his string quartets.

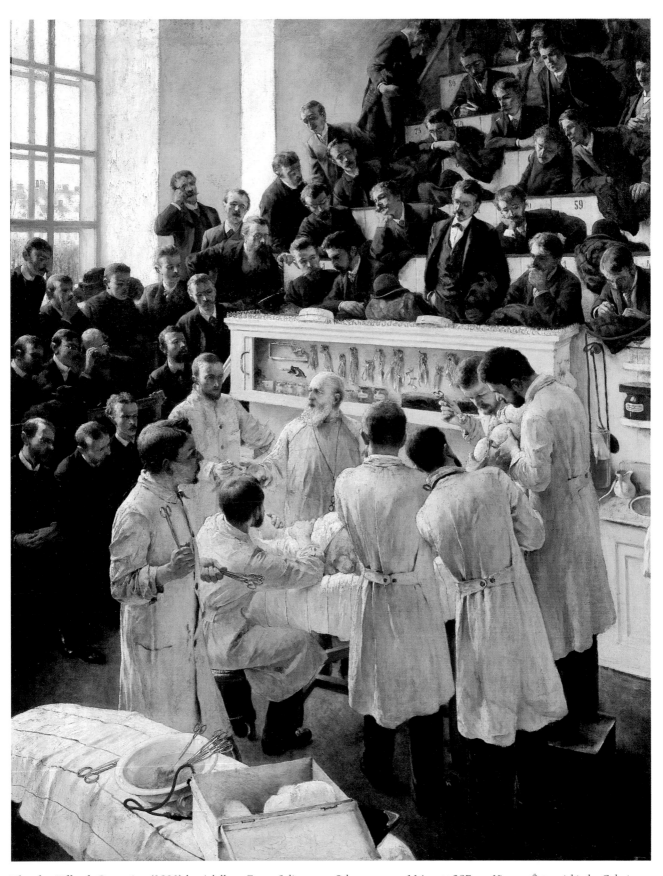

Theodor Billroth Operating (1890) by Adalbert Franz Seligmann. Oil on canvas, 114cm × 287cm. *Vienna, Österreichische Galerie Belvedere.*

44

Dr Péan Operating (1891–1892)

by Henri de Toulouse-Lautrec

Henri de Toulouse-Lautrec (1864–1901) is believed to have suffered from pyknodysostosis, a rare autosomal recessive disorder. Evidence supporting this idea is that he was of small stature with abnormally short limbs, he had a large skull associated with frontal bossing, he fractured both his legs in childhood and his parents were first cousins. Perhaps these deformities and his frequent contact with doctors in his early life accounted for his lifelong interest in the profession. In fact, he often said that if he had not been a painter he would have liked to have been a doctor. The reverse is true of the subject of this painting, Dr Jules Émile Péan (1830–1898). He was a distinguished French surgeon, but had at one time wanted to be a painter. Apart from the forceps that he invented (which were later modified by Spencer Wells), he is noted for having carried out the first gastric resection in 1879, although the patient died five days later, and the first successful elective splenectomy for cysts, and was one of the first to remove individual fibroids from the uterus rather than resorting to a total hysterectomy. The core of his work was summarized in his massive nine-volume *Leçons de clinique chirurgicale*.

In this painting, the surgeon appears to be carrying out a tonsillectomy (or possibly a tracheostomy). The artist has stressed the massive form of the surgeon engaged in delicate surgery, the remainder of the painting being much less detailed, and little more than background to the main event. But although general anaesthesia was now available and antiseptic surgery promoted by many, the surgeon here still wears his frock-coat with a white napkin around his neck. The view is a little obstructed by the head of an assistant on the right, just as it might have been in real life.

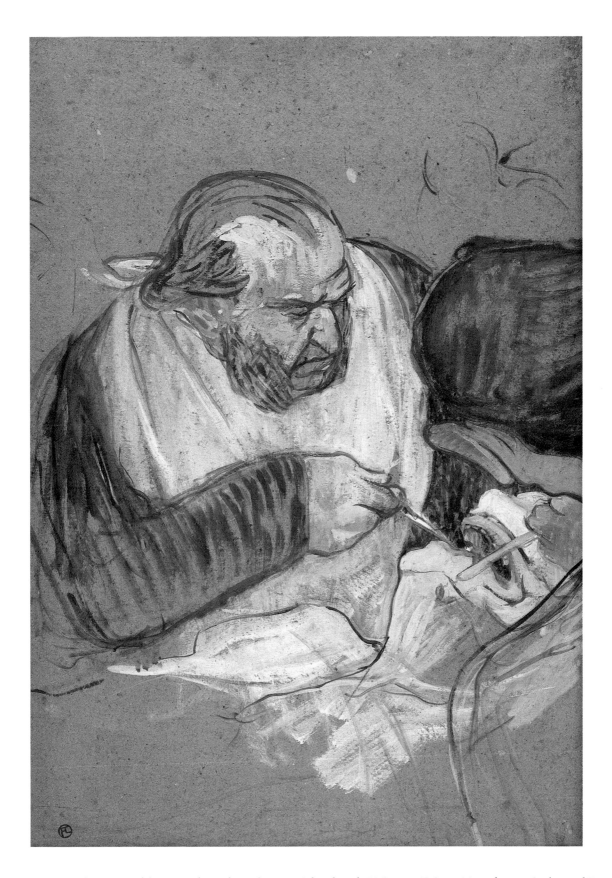

Dr Péan Operating (1891–1892) by Henri de Toulouse-Lautrec. Oil on board, 73.9 cm × 49.9 cm. *Massachusetts, Sterling and Francine Clark Art Institute.*

45

The Bad Doctors (1892)

by James Ensor

The patient's response to the surgeon or physician has attracted the attention of artists, particularly from the 16th century. Sometimes the patient's fear and dread is all too obvious, as is so evident in some of the early paintings depicting the surgeon at work. Some artists have portrayed the patient's acceptance of the inevitability of a fatal outcome. This was not uncommon in several Victorian paintings, such as *Doubtful Hope* by Frank Holl and *Sentence of Death* by John Collier. Of course, several notable artists of the Georgian period, such as Hogarth, Gillray and Cruikshank, while depicting the suffering of patients, at the same time poked fun at the profession, perhaps deservedly so in many cases. But this work by James Ensor (1860–1949) can hardly be considered humorous.

Ensor was born in Ostend of a British father and Flemish mother and seldom left the city. His early work was often criticized, but eventually he was considered a pioneer in the Expressionist movement, and was made a Baron in 1930. In his work he often produced biting caricatures of politicians, clergymen, judges and doctors, whom he saw as hypocritical, pompous and envious.

This work, painted when the artist was clinically depressed, is vitriolic and scathing of surgeons and physicians. A detailed analysis hardly seems necessary, because the images speak for themselves. The note in the foreground states that the patient has had a paracentesis and peritonitis has resulted. The patient is clearly very distressed.

Ensor played the harmonium and was a talented musician. It is said that he could play the flute when it was inserted up his nose! He was essentially a loner with a fear of crowds, and was highly strung and over-sensitive. He never married and in later life was looked after by two servants. Perhaps the painting reveals less about the profession than about the artist himself.

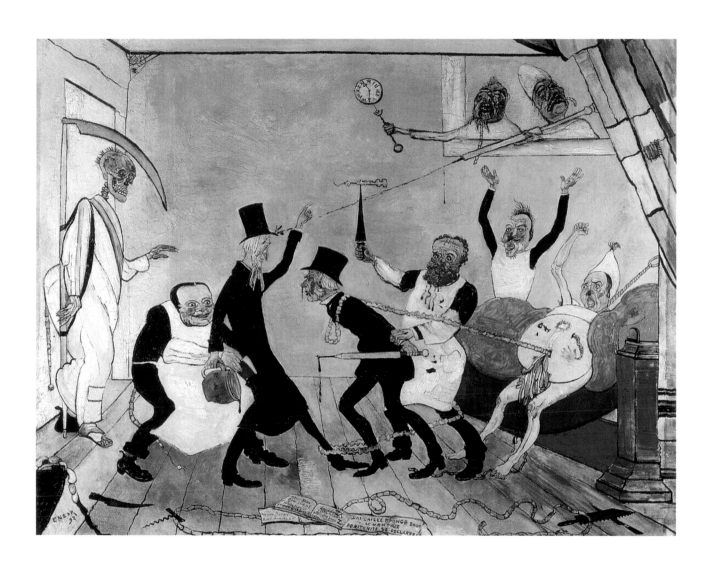

The Bad Doctors (1892) by James Ensor. Oil on panel, 50 cm × 61 cm. *Brussels, Université Libre de Bruxelles.*

46

An Exam at the Faculty of Medicine in Paris (1901)

by Henri de Toulouse-Lautrec

Toulouse-Lautrec came from an aristocratic professional family. His cousin and close friend Gabriel Tapié de Céleyran came to Paris in 1891 to begin an internship with Dr Jules Émile Péan (1830–1898), who we have seen was then a famous surgeon (Plate 44). Lautrec spent much time with his cousin at the hospital, becoming increasingly interested in the scenes and personalities he found there.

In this work, the artist commemorates Gabriel's oral examination in 1899 to be admitted to the Faculty. He is seen defending his thesis, *Sur un cas d'elytrocèle postérieure*, which he dedicated to Péan. He sits across the table from the board of examiners – the white-haired gentleman is Dr Jean Fournier, a famous venereologist and an expert on congenital syphilis, and the prominent figure facing the candidate is a Dr Robert Wurtz.

There are few paintings of doctors in training – one by the Russian painter Leonid Pasternak and one by the Puerto Rican artist Oller y Cestero, both in the Musée d'Orsay. This painting by Lautrec of a student being examined appears to be unique. The future of Dr Tapié is unknown, but we do know that Lautrec was by now a very sick man, suffering from the effects of alcoholism and syphilis. This was his last painting and he died the same year at the age of 36.

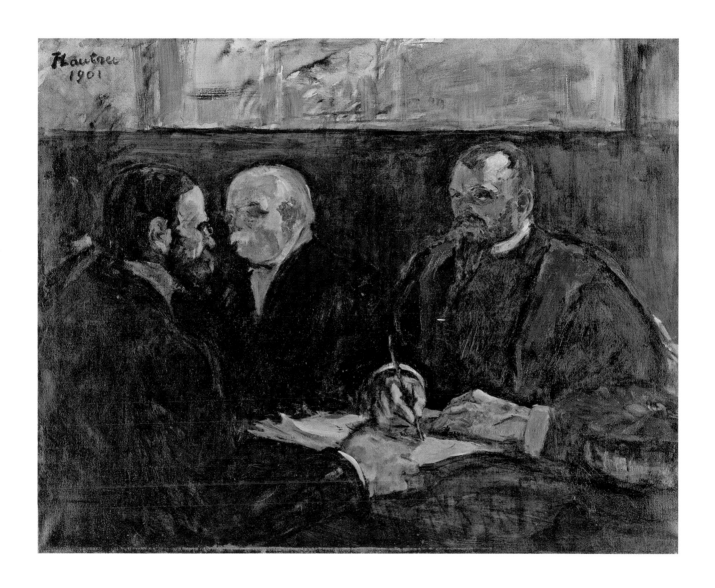

An Exam at the Faculty of Medicine in Paris (1901) by Henri de Toulouse-Lautrec. Oil on canvas, 65 cm × 81 cm. *Albi, Musée Toulouse-Lautrec.*

47

An Anxious Hour (1865)

by Fanny (Mrs Alexander F.) Farmer

Many artists have been attracted to the theme of the sick child and worried parents. For example, Dutch genre painters of the 17th century, including Gabriel Metsu and Pieter de Hooch, Norwegian artists, such as Christian Krohg and particularly Edvard Munch, the Finnish artist Helene Schjerfbeck, and the American artist Norman Rockwell have all painted the subject. But it was in Victorian England that the concept attracted the most attention, from artists such as Thomas Webster, Luke Fildes and several others, including, in this very sensitive painting of the subject, Fanny Farmer (fl 1855–1867), who exhibited under her husband's name as Mrs Alexander F. Farmer. The latter signature appears at the bottom of the work. Both her husband and sister-in-law were artists.

The work is particularly attractive because there is no mawkish sentimentality as in a number of Victorian paintings of the period. So many know the situation – the child is pale and languid, the orange slices remain untouched, the mother looks on with affection and concern. Even with all the treatments available nowadays, the scene still repeats itself, as for example in the works of Susan Macfarlane in the late 1990s (Plate 66).

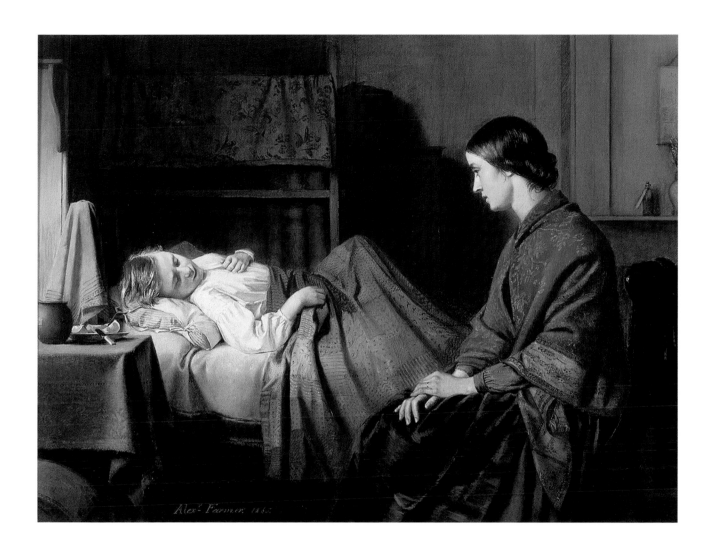

An Anxious Hour (1865) by Fanny (Mrs Alexander F.) Farmer. Oil on wood, 30.2 cm × 40.7 cm. *London, Victoria and Albert Picture Library.*

48

The Good Samaritan (1899)

by William Small

The 19th century produced many works of art that depicted the caring physician, often seen with a sick child. His diagnostic techniques, however, were very much limited to what he could see and hear, and very few effective treatments were available. There were, of course, no antibiotics. It is understandable therefore that the doctor's skills centred very much on his sympathetic understanding of the patient's problems – skills that in our present-day, technologically far more advanced society, sometimes seem to neglect.

In this typical example of the genre, the well-dressed doctor, a reflection of his social standing, has been summoned to see a sick child in a gypsy encampment. His carriage and driver are seen in the background. The stethoscope had been first introduced by Réné Laënnec in 1816 and the doctor is shown using the binaural instrument developed subsequently and considered a very important part of his armamentarium at the time the picture was painted.

William Small (1843–1929) was born in Edinburgh and studied at the Royal Scottish Academy, but eventually moved to London in 1865. He became well known at the time as a water-colourist, illustrator and also lithographer. He was very prolific and his illustrations appeared in many magazines and books, including Fielding's *Tom Jones*. This work is one of his rare oil paintings. And although the artist is little known nowadays, his *Good Samaritan* continues to attract interest, as it reflects society's image of the caring doctor at the time.

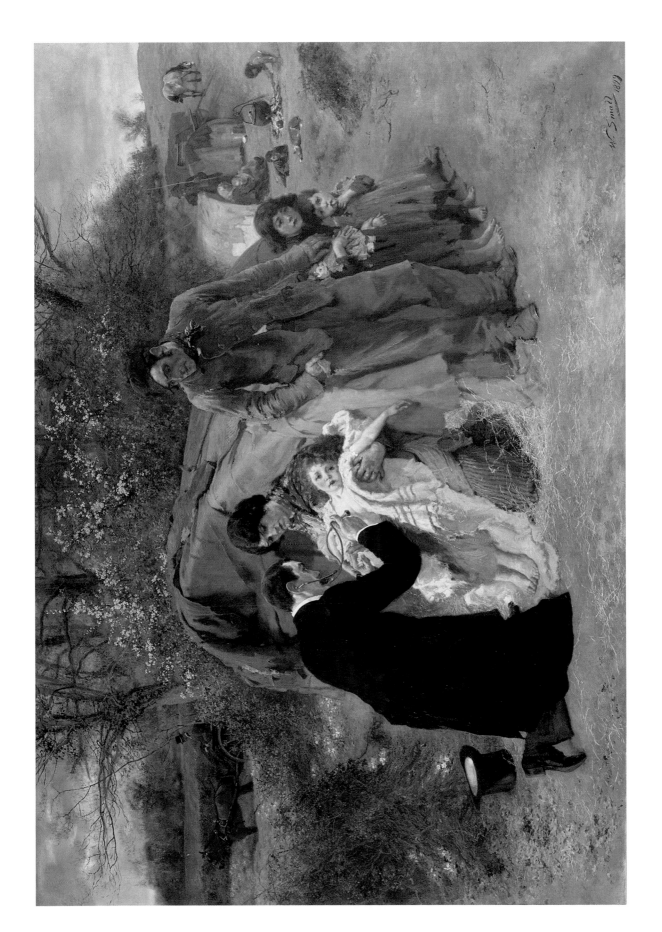

The Good Samaritan (1899) by William Small. *Oil on canvas, 159 cm × 245 cm. Leicester, New Walk Museum, Leicester City Museum Service.*

49

The First Trial of X-ray Therapy for Cancer of the Breast (1907–1908)

by Georges-Alexandre Chicotot

Several renowned surgeons have also been accomplished artists, including Sir Charles Bell, Sir Francis Haden, Henry Tonks and recently, Sir Roy Calne. But there have been very few practising physicians who at the same time were noted artists. Georges-Alexandre Chicotot, a French physician, is an exception. He first graduated from the École des Beaux-Arts in Paris and then, in 1899, the École du Médecine. He subsequently became Head of Radiotherapy at the Hôpital Broca. He painted several works of medical interest, including *Le Tubage* (1904), *Une Autopsie* (1905) and this later work. Here, he depicts himself wearing a top hat and white apron, as was customary for doctors working in their laboratory at the time. He is seen carrying out the first trial of X-ray therapy for breast cancer. He holds a watch to time the exposure, in his other hand he holds a sort of Bunsen burner to heat the vessel holding the Crookes tube generator. The X-rays are focused on the affected breast by a glass cylinder and the apparatus on the mantelpiece is an electrical transformer.

William Halsted (1852–1922) of Johns Hopkins Hospital is noted for having advocated total mastectomy for breast cancer in the 1890s, and this was soon widely accepted. This was a very disfiguring operation, which by the 1960s was found to be unnecessary and was replaced by a more conservative operation followed by radiation, originally advocated by Geoffrey Keynes of St Bartholomew's Hospital in the 1930s. Following on from the pioneering research of Marie and Pierre Curie and Henri Becquerel, in 1904 it was shown that radium destroyed diseased cells, which led to the use of radiation treatment for cancer. This painting by Chicotot therefore shows one of the very early attempts to treat breast cancer with X-rays – although clearly the artist as well as others at the time had not fully realized the harmful effects of X-rays to themselves, as he is not protecting himself in any way.

Chicotot received a number of awards during his lifetime, including a bronze medal at the World Exhibition and later a Légion d'Honneur in 1922 and another medal from the Academy of Medicine for his work on X-rays.

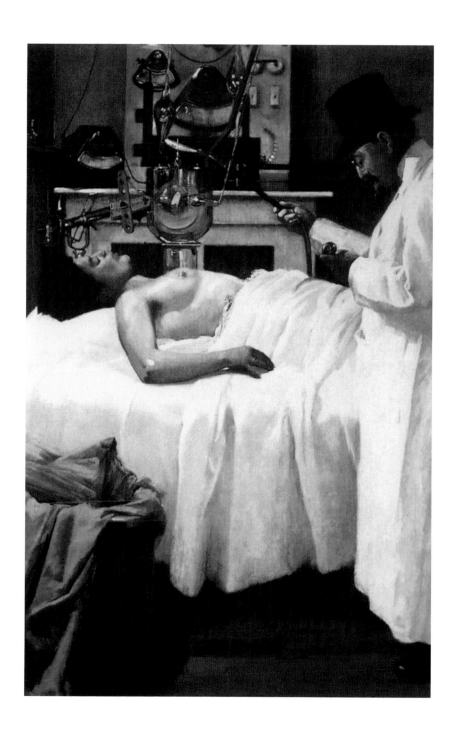

The First Trial of X-ray Therapy for Cancer of the Breast (1907–1908) by Georges-Alexandre Chicotot. ? Oil on canvas, *Paris, Musée de l'Assistance Publique–Hôpitaux de Paris.*

50

Ablutions (1932)

by Sir Stanley Spencer

The artists included in this series of essays are occasionally physicians or patients themselves, but more often are observers of treatment. Here, not only was the artist a perceptive observer but he was also involved in the care of war-wounded. Sir Stanley Spencer (1891–1959) first trained at the Slade School of Art in London, but in 1915 enlisted in the Royal Army Medical Corps, where he served first as an orderly and then, in 1916 and until the end of the war, with the Field Ambulance in Macedonia. These experiences affected him greatly and formed the basis for a series of murals and paintings now at the Sandham Memorial Chapel at Burghclere, near Newbury. Louis and Mary Behrend built this private chapel as a memorial to their friend's brother, Lieutenant Henry Willoughby Sandham, who had died in the war. They commissioned Spencer to do a series of murals for the chapel based on the artist's memories of active service.

In this particular work from the Chapel, he has depicted the subject of soldiers carrying out their daily ablutions. Some of the men are drying themselves as well as each other, and one is washing his hair. The main character, however, is having his body painted with iodine. Iodine had had many uses in the past, but, according to Martindale's *Extra Pharmacopoeia*, its main use then was as an antiseptic, particularly for disinfecting the skin prior to a surgical operation, and for the treatment of open and infected wounds, although in this latter regard, by the time of the Second World War, it would be replaced by acriflavine. In this illustration, it seems more likely that iodine was being used not for its antiseptic qualities but rather for its parasiticidal action and for cases of ringworm of the scalp and body, medical conditions relatively common among soldiers serving in the First World War. Incidentally, while all this is going on, one orderly is busily polishing the taps. It seems that soldiers have always been involved with 'spit and polish', no matter what the circumstances may be!

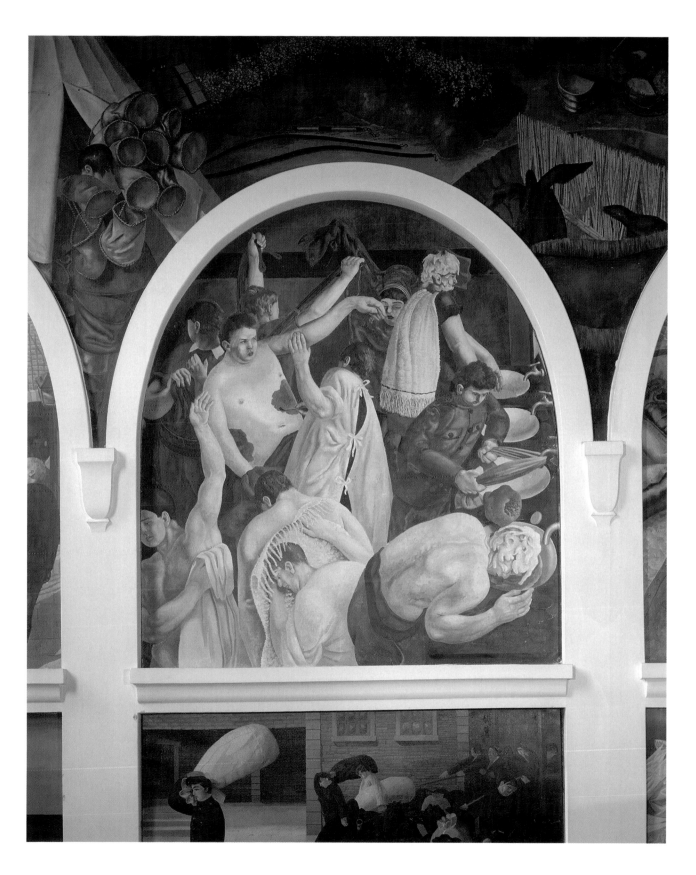

Ablutions (1932) by Sir Stanley Spencer. Oil on canvas, 213.4 cm × 185.4 cm. Burghclere, Sandham Memorial Chapel.
© National Trust Photo Library, © Estate of Stanley Spencer 2005. All rights reserved, DACS.

51

Travoys Arriving with Wounded at a Dressing Station at Smol, Macedonia, September 1916 (1919)

by Sir Stanley Spencer

This work by Sir Stanley Spencer refers to events probably later than the preceding work, when he was with the field ambulance in Macedonia from 1916–1918. Although he was appointed an official war artist in 1918, his experiences found their most memorable expression later and formed a series of murals for the Sandham Memorial Chapel.

Spencer volunteered for the Field Ambulance in August 1916 and was posted to Macedonia. A year later he became an infantryman in the 7th Battalion of the Royal Berkshire Regiment, where he served in the Balkans until the end of 1918. One of the works based on this service is *Travoys Arriving with Wounded at a Dressing Station at Smol, Macedonia, September 1916*: a travoy was a sort of sledge with one end being attached to the horse's harness, while the other dragged on the ground. The injured are all seriously ill, lying wrapped up in blankets, one being consoled by an orderly. In the background the military surgeons can be seen operating on one of the wounded.

The surgeons would have been officers in the Royal Army Medical Corps, which had been set up in 1898. The Royal Army Medical College, in Netley, for instructing medical officers was opened four years later. The RAMC thereafter had its own uniform and usual ranks and titles. Those with a basic medical qualification entered the Corps with at least the rank of full lieutenant; specialists were given more senior ranks. The RAMC also had its own badge with the characteristic medical motif of a staff entwined with a snake and the motto *In arduis fidelis*. Incidentally, the US Army Medical Corps has a similar badge, but with two snakes!

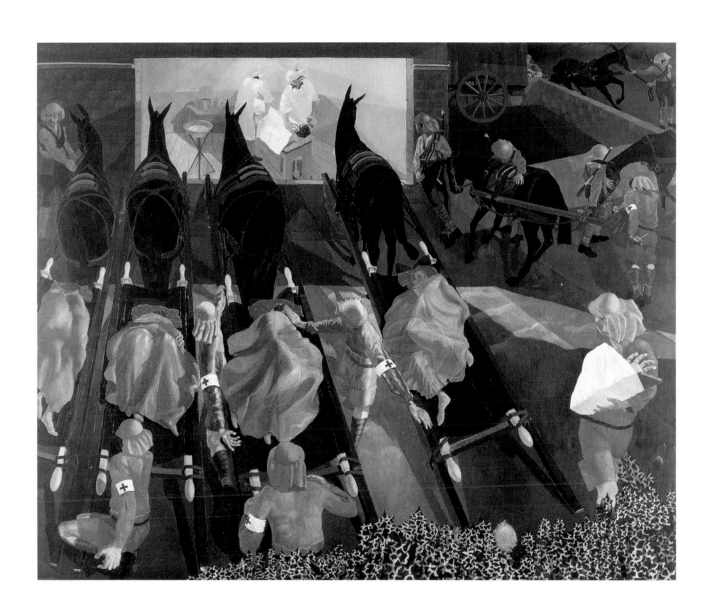

Travoys Arriving with Wounded at a Dressing Station at Smol, Macedonia, September 1916 (1919) by Sir Stanley Spencer. Oil on canvas, 180 cm × 215 cm. *London, Imperial War Museum, London, The Bridgeman Art Library.*

52

Dr Hans Koch, the Dermatologist and Urologist (1921)

by Otto Dix

The artist Otto Dix (1891–1969), like other German artists of the same period, such as George Grosz and Max Beckmann, expressed much of their resentment with their post-war country in their art. Dix depicted the decadence of society, especially in relation to sex. Having trained at the Dresden School of Arts and Crafts, he enlisted in the German Army in 1914. After the war he was invited to Düsseldorf by Hans Koch, a doctor and art collector. Dix was described at the time as somewhat of a dandy and ladies' man and a superb dancer. This made a great impression on Koch's wife, Martha. Around this time, Dr Koch commissioned Dix to do his portrait. The Koch's marriage was already in crisis, and eventually Otto Dix and Martha became lovers, and Koch divorced his wife two years later. She then married Dix.

As we shall see in another, but later, portrait by Dix (Plate 59), the background was important in defining the character of the subject. He commented himself that with regard to the sitter's external appearance '… even the folds of the clothing, the person's posture, his hands and ears, immediately tell the painter something about the model's inner being … The outside of things is [also] important to me, because depicting external appearance allows one simultaneously to capture the inner being at the same time'. This is all very clear in this portrait of Dr Hans Koch.

Dr Koch was described as both 'a dermatologist and urologist'. All the trappings of his surgery are included in the background. One wonders whether he might have been a venereologist, in view of the nature of some of the instruments. Dr Koch himself is certainly not portrayed as an attractive person, which may well have been the artist's intention given the relationship he had with the sitter's wife. Many German students at the time belonged to fencing fraternities (Schlage Verbindungen) and perhaps the scars on Dr Koch's cheek are the result of duelling. These societies and the artist's work were both condemned by the Nazis. From this painting much can be learnt of the sitter and of the artist's opinion of his subject – very different from the orthodox formal portraits of many physicians and surgeons.

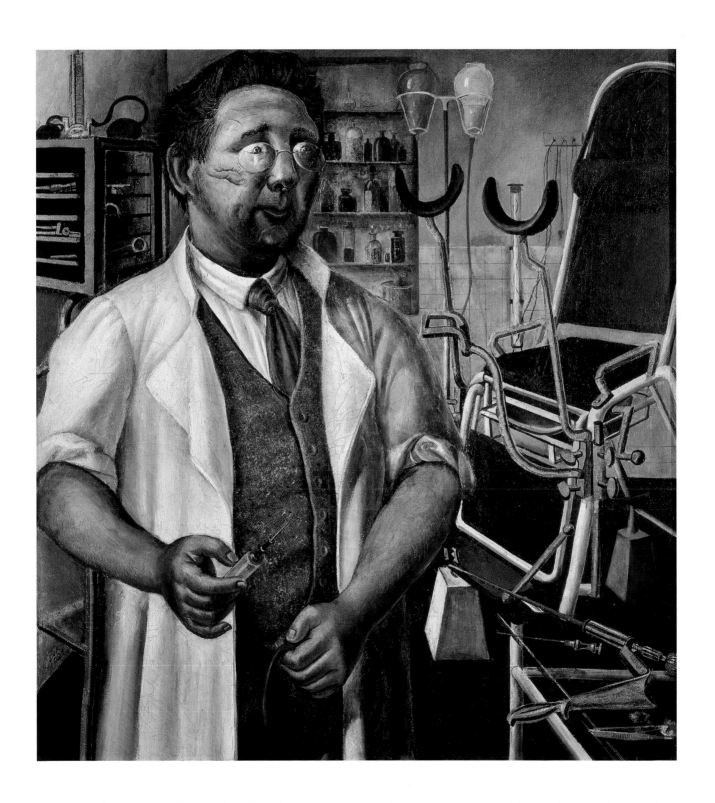

Dr Hans Koch, the Dermatologist and Urologist (1921) by Otto Dix. Oil on canvas, 100.5 cm × 90 cm. *Köln, Rheinisches Bildarchiv.*

53

The Cardiologist, H. Vaquez, and his Assistant (1926)

by Édouard Vuillard

Édouard Vuillard (1868–1940) was another artist, like Toulouse-Lautrec, with an interest in the profession. He was a French artist who was deeply attached to his widowed mother and never married. He trained at the École des Beaux-Arts and later the Académie Julien in Paris. He became particularly regarded for his paintings of keenly observed interiors and subjects. Vuillard befriended and painted several established medical figures, including the surgeon Dr Antonin Gosset and the cardiologist Louis Henri Vaquez (1860–1936), of whom he painted at least two portraits, including this one. At the time of his death Vaquez was an outstanding physician. Early in his career he began to specialize in the developing subject of cardiology and his *Diseases of the Heart* was widely admired and was translated into English in 1924. William Osler, in 1903, thought that the disease of polycythaemia with cyanosis was a new entity, but later acknowledged that Vaquez had described it earlier in 1892, and in the English-speaking world it became referred to as Vaquez-Osler disease. Vaquez also studied cardiac arrhythmias and was one of the first cardiologists in France to employ electrocardiography. He also invented an instrument referred to as a 'sphygmotensiophone', apparently to study blood pressure, which was possibly a modification of the existing sphygmograph for recording pulse waves. In this painting, Vaquez's assistant, Dr Parvu, is on the right, attending to the machine.

Vaquez was not only an eminent cardiologist but also a connoisseur of art, and owned works by Vuillard and also by Toulouse-Lautrec, Rodin, Renoir, Degas and Redon. These were probably presented to him for his professional services by his often wealthy and fashionable clients. He was, for example, the principal heart doctor to the young Marcel Proust and his mother.

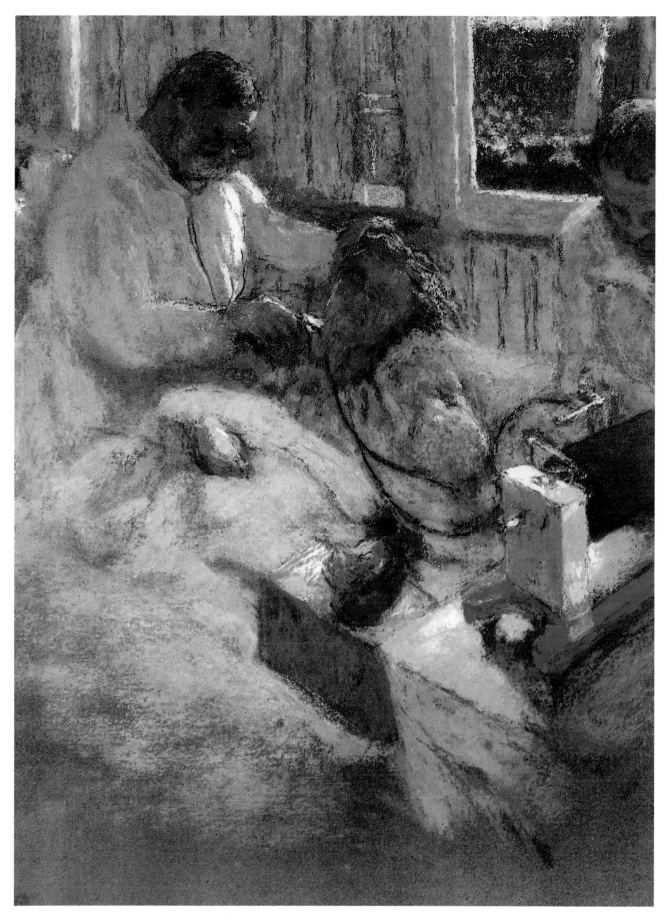

The Cardiologist, H. Vaquez, and his Assistant (1926) by Édouard Vuillard. Pastel and glue-based distemper, 65 cm × 50 cm. *Paris, Musée de l'Assistance Publique–Hôpitaux de Paris.*

54

The Operation (1929)
by Christian Schad

Christian Schad (1894–1982) was a German artist who, around 1918 while living in Geneva, began to experiment with photography. This led him a few years later to adopt a very realistic style referred to as *Neue Sachlichkeit* (New Objectivity), with clear, detailed, highly realistic paintings and drawings. Many of his works expressed his disillusionment with post-war Germany, like several other artists at the time, most notably Otto Dix, George Grosz and Max Beckmann. Unlike these artists, however, Schad did not employ caricature but coolly depicted every realistic detail of his subjects and surroundings. It is for this reason that this work is of special interest here.

One evening at a dinner party, Schad befriended Dr Haustein, a surgeon who was on call. When he was called to the hospital for a case of acute appendicitis, he invited the artist to accompany him into the operating theatre, and had him gowned as his colleague. Schad was greatly impressed and fascinated by the way in which the surgical team worked so closely together with almost clockwork precision. Schad then returned to his studio to make a painting based on his sketches. When the surgeon saw his work, he was so interested that he brought a number of surgical instruments to the studio for the artist to copy in order to add authenticity. However, the surgeon thought the colour of the intestines was too pale: 'You have concentrated too much on the anatomy, you must see living intestines'. When subsequently the artist witnessed a Caesarean operation, he found that he could not recognize any detail with so much blood. It was much less interesting to him than the almost bloodless appendicectomy. In this painting, the operation appears not to be conducted under general anaesthesia. Local and spinal anaesthesia had been introduced in the 1890s.

The history of appendicitis is interesting. Until the end of the 19th century, the main cause of pain in the lower right quadrant was attributed to disease of the caecum and appendix, referred to as perityphlitis. But it gradually became clear that the culprit was the appendix. Charles McBurney, in 1889, described 'McBurney's point' as the site of maximum tenderness over the inflamed appendix. Lawson Tait was the first British surgeon to diagnose acute appendicitis and to treat it with removal of the appendix in 1880, but only reported it in detail 10 years later. And in 1902, Sir Frederick Treves successfully operated on King Edward VII for appendicitis, or perhaps more accurately, to drain an appendix abscess. Thus Schad's painting clearly illustrates how far surgery for appendicitis had progressed, becoming almost routine in just under 30 years.

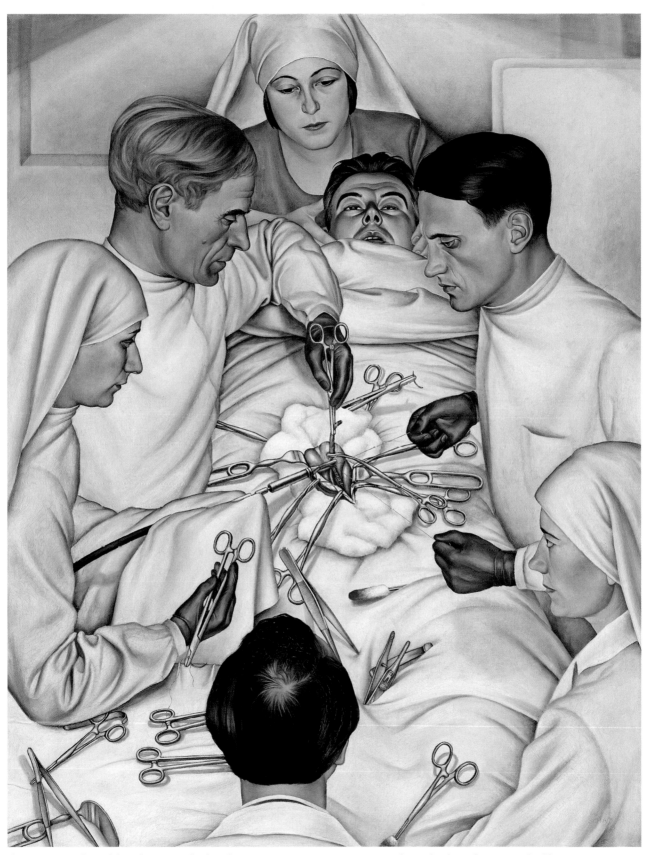

The Operation (1929) by Christian Schad. Oil on canvas, 125 cm × 95 cm. *Munich, Städtische Galerie im Lenbachhaus.*
© Christian Schad Stiftung Aschaffenburg/VG Bild-Kunst, Bonn and DACS, London 2005.

55

The Fever Van (1935)

by L. S. Lowry

Both Helen Bradley (1900–1979) and Laurence Stephen Lowry (1887–1976) became renowned for their depiction in their paintings of Lancashire life. But whereas Helen Bradley's work largely relates to her childhood experiences in middle-class Edwardian society, Lowry's paintings essentially concern working-class life in a slightly later period. And whereas Bradley's work has a childlike fairytale attraction, Lowry's work is renowned for its stark and realistic depiction of the poverty and working life of the time.

Lowry portrayed several subjects of medical interest, including *A Doctor's Waiting Room* (c 1920), *An Accident* (1926), *The Cripples* (1949), *Ancoats Hospital Outpatients' Hall* (1952) and the one reproduced here, *The Fever Van* (1935).

As a child growing up in Lancashire in the 1930s, one of us (AEHE) remembers only too well the fear tinged with morbid curiosity that the arrival of a fever van engendered among neighbours. The 'fever van' was a colloquial term for the ambulance that transported patients with an infectious disease to the local infectious diseases hospital for isolation. This was usually diphtheria or scarlet fever, for which at the time there was no specific treatment and for which the morbidity and mortality were high. All the possessions and toys of the patient, almost always a young child, would be destroyed and the house totally disinfected from floor to ceiling and fumigated. The disruption to the household was considerable and there was a high probability that the child might never return home but die in hospital.

Lowry has captured the atmosphere surrounding the arrival of the fever van with the use of dark images and sombre colours of the terraced houses, the outline of a church tower in the background and the ubiquitous smoking chimney. The clustering of onlookers and the terraced housing reflect the overcrowding of the time – an important factor in the spread of scarlet fever and diphtheria.

The fever van became relegated to history by the 1950s and nowadays, as a result of immunization (for diphtheria), antibiotics and better housing conditions, diphtheria and scarlet fever are far less common and much less severe than formerly.

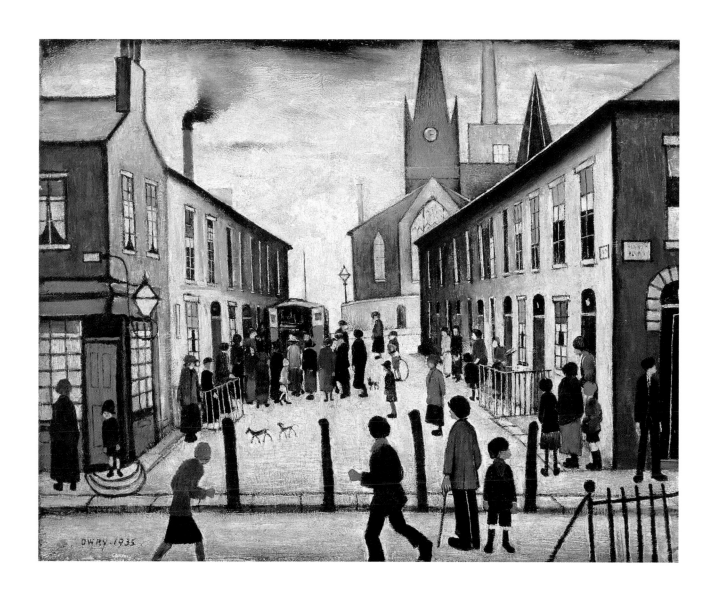

The Fever Van (1935) by L. S. Lowry. Oil on canvas, 43.1 cm × 53.3 cm. *Liverpool, National Museums Liverpool (Walker Art Gallery).*

56

Dr Louis Viau (1936–1937)

by Édouard Vuillard

By the time Édouard Vuillard (1868–1940) had painted this picture in 1936–1937, dentistry had come a very long way from the days of the itinerant tooth-puller. The subject is surrounded by the equipment of his profession, including an X-ray machine and an electrically operated tooth drill, although at the time many dentists outside the main cities would still have often been using foot-operated drills. General and local anaesthesia would now be widely available.

The subject of the painting is a Dr Louis Viau, whose portrait in his dental office Vuillard had also painted in 1914. By now, in his late 60s, Dr Viau has done very well, surrounded as he is by shelves crammed with books and objets d'art, in a luxurious office on the Boulevard Haussmann. But the artist seems more concerned with presenting the image of the technical side of the speciality. He may have been more than a little amused by the dental surgeon's pose than intimidated by him. Few could turn a visit to a dentist into a mysteriously warm and interesting experience as the artist has done here.

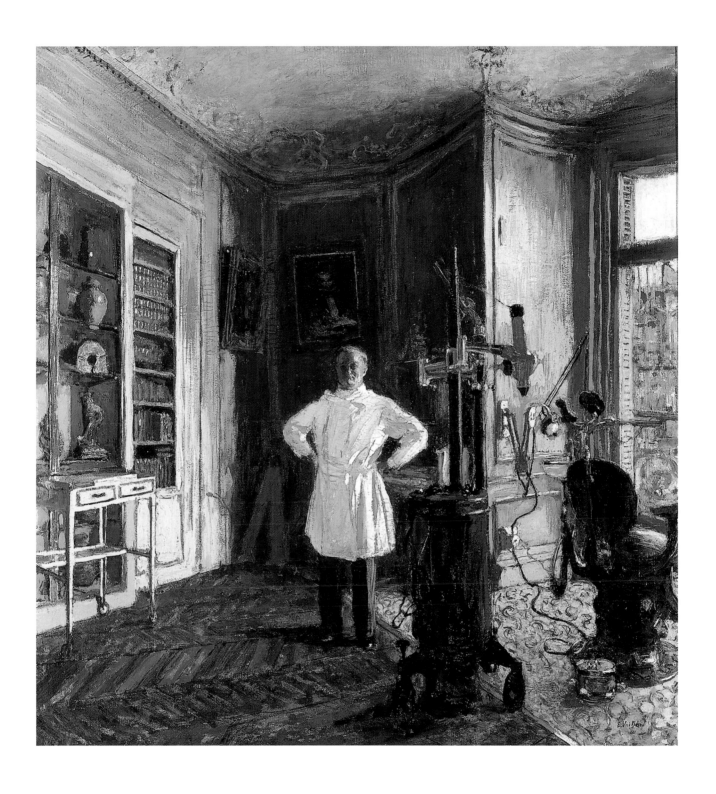

Dr Louis Viau (1936–1937) by Édouard Vuillard. Distemper on canvas, 88 cm × 81 cm. *Paris, Musée d'Orsay.*
© Photo RMN, © Hervé Lewandowski.

57

'I Waxes and I Wanes, Sir' (1944)

by Mervyn Peake

Mervyn Peake (1911–1968) was raised in China, the son of a missionary doctor. From an early age he demonstrated a real gift for drawing and in later life became a talented artist as well as a writer and poet.

In his life he was somewhat unconventional. He was in many ways a loner, and his behaviour, while serving in the Army during the Second World War, attracted much criticism and exasperation from his superiors. At this time he began to suffer from insomnia, depression and irritability, and in 1942, he was released from military service on medical grounds. A few years later he developed a progressive neurodegenerative disease characterized by mental confusion, loss of memory, a tremor and visual hallucinations, which he portrayed in several sketches. This very debilitating disease necessitated his full-time confinement to various psychiatric centres for the last four years of his life.

He saw many physicians and neurologists for an explanation of his symptoms, including Roger Gilliat at the National Hospital, Queen's Square, London. He had a number of investigations and various trials of treatment, including electroconvulsive therapy (which he most feared). No specific diagnosis, however, was ever made and no effective treatment was offered.

Like many patients in a similar situation, he became frustrated and angry with the inability of the profession to find a diagnosis and treatment. This is demonstrated in this illustration from one of his books, ostensibly for children but clearly with a wider message.

The accompanying poem reads:

> 'I waxes, and I wanes, sir;
> I ebbs's and I flows;
> Some say it be my Brains, sir,
> Some says it be my Nose.
>
> It isn't as I'm slow, sir,
> (To cut a story long),
> It's just I'd *love* to know, sir,
> Which one of them is *wrong*.'

With hindsight and with improvements in our understanding of neurodegenerative diseases in recent years, the consensus is that Mervyn Peake probably suffered from dementia with Lewy bodies, for which there still remains no long-term effective treatment.

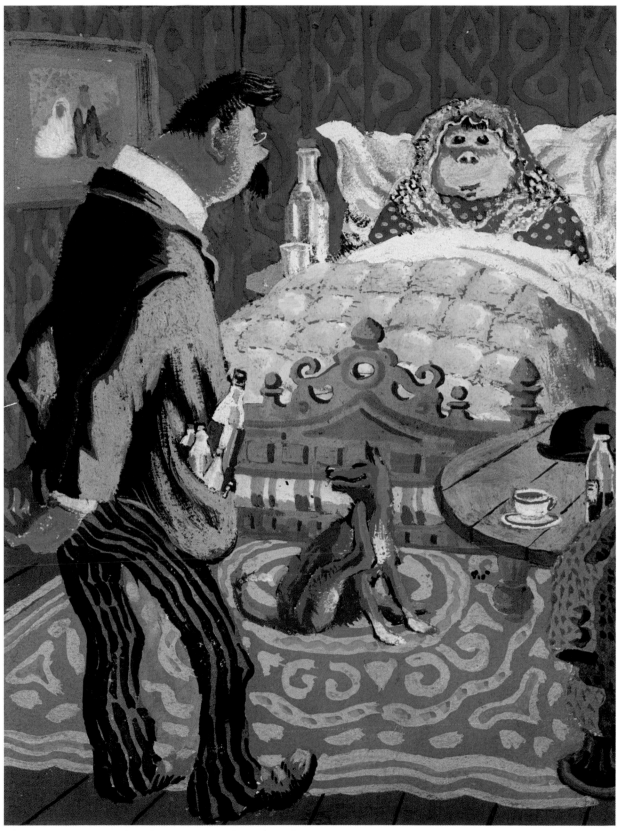

I Waxes, and I Wanes, Sir (1944) by Mervyn Peake. Colour illustration, 23.1 cm × 17.7 cm *From:* Rhymes without Reason, *London: Eyre & Spottiswoode, 1944.*
Poem and artwork with kind permission of the Estate of Mervyn Peake.

58

The Microscope (1948)
by Dame Barbara Hepworth

A number of specialized branches of surgery have evolved and benefited from technology. This is well illustrated in the case of otological surgery. The operation of fenestration was designed to create an alternative window, or fenestra, into the inner ear, so bypassing the footplate of the stapes that had become fixed due to otosclerosis. The first successful attempt is credited to Adolf Passow (1859–1926) of Heidelberg in 1897, but refinements were necessary and these were achieved by a number of surgeons over the following years, most notably by E. R. Garnett Passe (1904–1952), who published a refined and successful technique in 1939. Over the remainder of his short life, he performed over one thousand such operations, which were made much easier using a binocular dissecting microscope, as depicted in this work by Barbara Hepworth.

Dame Barbara Hepworth (1903–1975) was a well-known sculptor who, in 1939, moved to St Ives in Cornwall. She remained there for the rest of her life – her studio becoming a mecca for the many interested in her work. Sarah, the third of triplets born to the artist, developed osteomyelitis and in this way Barbara Hepworth befriended the orthopaedic surgeon Norman Capener, the consultant in the subject at the Princess Elizabeth Orthopaedic Hospital in Exeter, who looked after Sarah. Barbara Hepworth recalled that around 1947, a suggestion was made that she might like to watch an operation. She became completely fascinated by the experience, '... the extraordinary beauty of purpose and co-ordination between human beings all dedicated to the saving of life, and the way that unity of idea and purpose dictated a perfection of concentration, movement and gesture ...', – not dissimilar from the German artist Christian Schad's response to seeing a surgical operation some years earlier (Plate 54). It also appealed to the sculptor in Hepworth.

Over a period of time, she created a number of works depicting various surgical operations, including the use of a microscope in a fenestration by Garnett Passe, as well as a variety of orthopaedic procedures by Norman Capener. In all, Barbara Hepworth produced over sixty hospital drawings and paintings, some of which have been reproduced and discussed in detail by John Booth FRCS, himself a former consultant ENT surgeon (*Journal of Laryngology & Otology* vol. 114, Suppl. 26, April 2000).

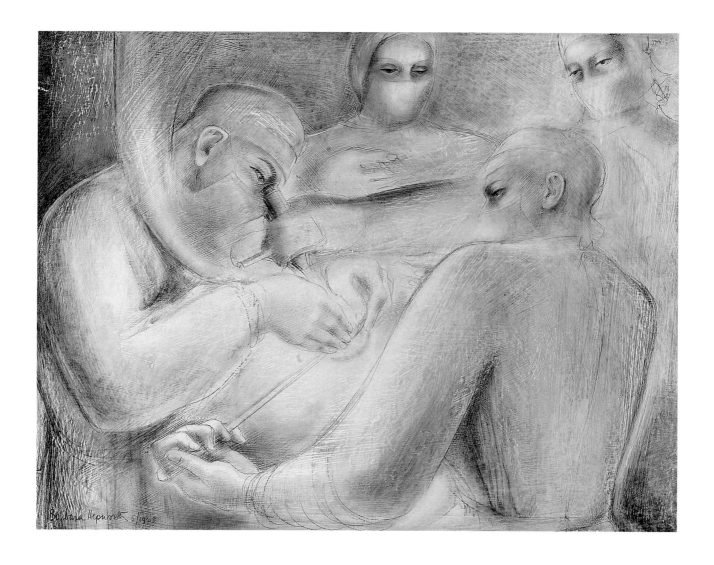

The Microscope (1948) by Dame Barbara Hepworth. Pencil and oil on gesso-prepared board, 54.6 cm × 70.3 cm.
© Bowness, Hepworth Estate.

59

Portrait of Dr Fritz Perls
(Founder of Gestalt Therapy) (1966)

by Otto Dix

Otto Dix was born in 1891 in Thuringia and came from a working-class family. Because of his social background, some commentators have concluded that he was perhaps motivated by political ideology. But in fact he remained throughout his life indifferent to politics and more concerned with being a realist and depicting life and events as he witnessed them.

Much of his art, of the 1920s, reflects the devastating and traumatic effects of trench warfare following his experiences as a sergeant at the front line in the war. After demobilization and further art training in Düsseldorf, he was eventually appointed Professor at the Dresden Academy. His war paintings were then succeeded by depictions of the decadence of German society at the time: feverish night-life and prostitution. In 1933, he was condemned by the Nazis for what they considered 'degenerate' art, and he left for Lake Constance, where he remained until his death in 1969.

From a medical point of view, he painted several very realistic depictions of disorders, including *The Lunatic* (1925), *Nude (Albino) Girl on a Fur* (1932) and many on the effects of aging. He also painted revealing portraits of contemporary doctors, including Dr Hans Koch (1921), a dermatologist and urologist (Plate 52), and Dr Mayer-Hermann (1926), a throat specialist, in both cases the backgrounds giving clues to the individual's professional interests. In all his many portraits, in fact, the chosen background adds to the meaning of the painting. He noted himself: 'Every person has his own special colour which affects the entire picture'.

In this painting of Dr Fritz Perls, the artist has used vibrant colours that add to the intense thoughtful gaze of the doctor. With his companion and co-worker Laura Perls, he founded the Gestalt School of psychotherapy. The aim of their approach was to consider the individual as a whole: the interaction between the individual and the environment with emphasis on the present rather than the past. Dix seems to have captured the intensity of the enquiring psychiatrist who is attempting to determine the underlying causes of a patient's problems.

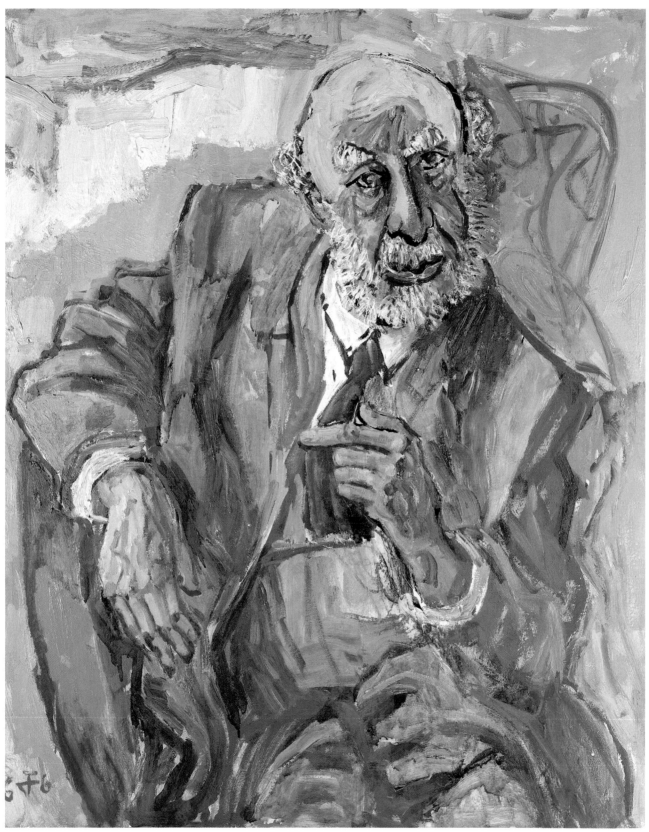

Portrait of Dr Fritz Perls (Founder of Gestalt Therapy) (1966) by Otto Dix. Oil and tempera on wood, 93 cm × 75 cm. *Liechtenstein, Otto Dix Foundation.*
© DACS 2005.

60

Tobacco Rose (1965)

by Mel Ramos

Up until the 1950s and 1960s, cigarette manufacturers often advertised their products by emphasizing associations with the 'good life', or with manliness, hardy and rugged; some brands appealed to feelings of loneliness, '... you're never alone with a ...'. There were even appeals to their supposed medical value. One American brand, *Spud*, recommended its value in colds and nose and throat congestion. One famous make claimed it was preferred by doctors.

The first major medical paper suggesting a link between smoking and lung cancer was published by F. H. Müller in Germany in 1939. Such a study had been generated, at least in part, by the Nazi cult of physical fitness – Hitler himself was a non-smoker and abhorred the habit. But it was the UK Medical Research Council, in 1947, that commissioned Austin Bradford Hill (1897–1991) and Richard Doll (1912–2005) to analyse the possible cause of the increasing mortality from lung cancer. Their first papers showing the relationship with smoking, appeared in the early 1950s, followed subsequently by many confirmatory studies.

But early on, not all were convinced of a causative relationship. Some suggested that the important factor was the personality of the smoker, some the paper used in the manufacture of cigarettes and some even the type of material used to light cigarettes. But by 1962, the Royal College of Physicians, and two years later the US Surgeon General's Advisory Committee, announced unequivocally that smoking causes lung cancer and later that it causes other serious diseases, including bronchitis and emphysema, as well as circulatory and cardiovascular disorders.

Although cigarette smoking is decreasing along with the incidence of lung cancer, worryingly, many young women take up the habit, in part in the belief that it creates a powerful image and as an aid to slimming. This particular painting personifies and thereby ridicules this belief.

The artist Mel Ramos (b 1935) studied at Sacramento State College. He subsequently became associated with Pop Art, a movement that began in the 1950s and uses imagery of mass culture in opposition to the intellectual culture of fine art. As here, Ramos often uses real figures against commercial products: an attractive and smiling young lady against a background of a trademark or similar. Here, this device cleverly mocks those who associate attractiveness with cigarette smoking.

But although the evidence for smoking causing lung cancer is now totally accepted, a number of questions still remain. Why, for example, may some lifelong smokers never develop lung cancer and why does the disease sometimes occur in lifelong non-smokers? One presumes that genetic factors may be involved.

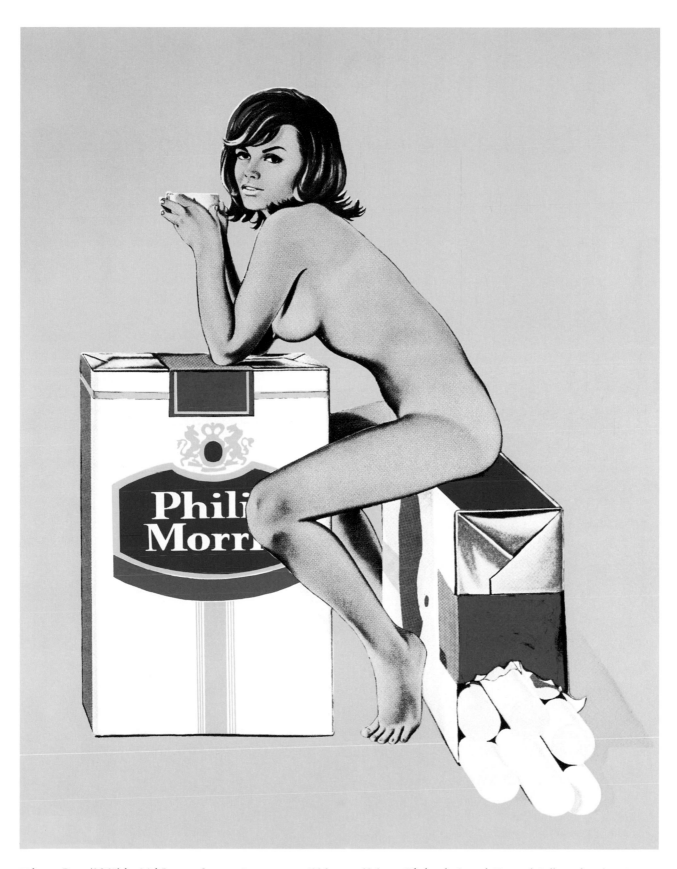

Tobacco Rose (1965) by Mel Ramos. Screenprint on paper, 76.2 cm × 60.9 cm. *Edinburgh, Scottish National Gallery of Modern Art.* © Mel Ramos.

61

Therapy *or* The Neuromuscular Clinic (1972)
by Murray Tod

There have been several artists who have depicted their impressions of their own doctor in practice – for example Goya's painting of Dr Arrieta, Richard Dadd's of Sir Alexander Morison (Plate 34), Norman Rockwell's of his family doctor, Dame Barbara Hepworth's of the surgeons Garnett Passe and Norman Capener, Andrew Wyeth's of the paediatrician Dr Margaret Handy, John Bellany's of Sir Roy Calne and Georges Chicotot's of himself (Plate 49).

This work by Murray Tod is the artist's light-hearted impression of AEHE's clinic for patients with neuromuscular disorders. It would be quite reasonable, as the artist has, to imagine that any outsider confronted with a hospital environment could be intimidated and perhaps overwhelmed by the variety of technologies. Here, we have various pieces of equipment for determining muscle power and for electromyography and nerve conduction studies. Even a hint of some bizarre therapies! He himself had been diagnosed as having a neuromuscular disease.

Murray Macpherson Tod (1909–1974) was born in Glasgow and trained at the Glasgow School of Art, and later the Royal College of Art. He left to work at the British School in Rome in 1935. He returned to Scotland before the war, after which he spent the rest of his life teaching art and etching and as a freelance artist. He exhibited widely, including at the Royal Academy and the Royal Scottish Academy, and was elected to several professional organizations, including the Royal Society of Painters and Etchers and the Royal Society of Arts. This work – really more a cartoon – provides a treasured memory of a wonderful artist, patient and friend with a great sense of humour.

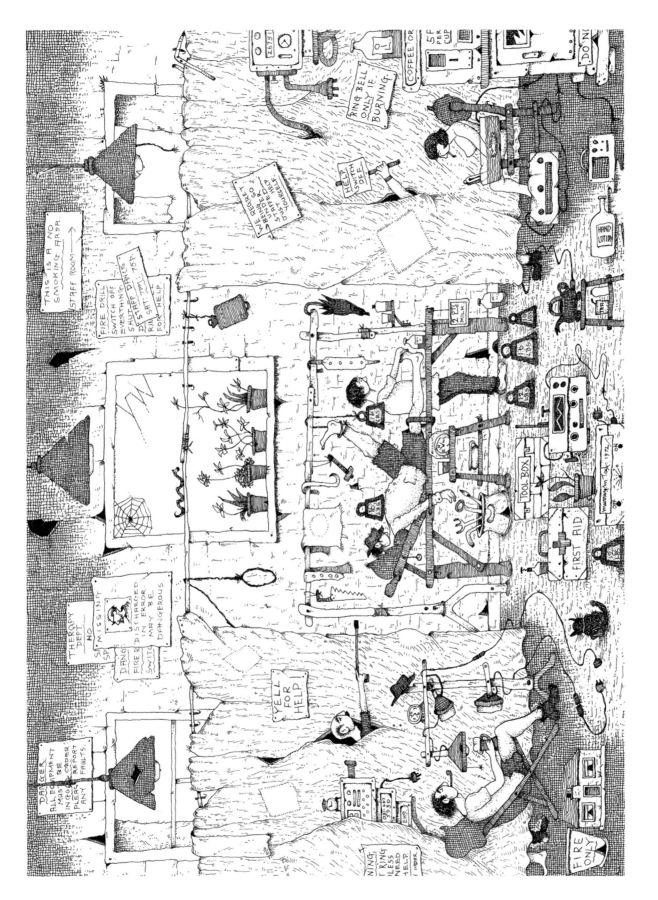

Therapy or *The Neuromuscular Clinic* (1972) by Murray Tod. Pen and ink and wash on paper, 39 cm × 55 cm. *Author's private collection.*

62

English Landscape with a Disruptive Gene (1987)

by Steven Campbell

Steven Campbell was born in Glasgow in 1953. From 1970 to 1977 he had a job in a steel works and then entered Glasgow School of Art. He graduated in 1982 with numerous prizes, including a Fulbright Scholarship that took him to New York, where he stayed until 1986, before returning to Scotland. In 1990, he was Artist in Residence in Sydney, Australia.

In studying the artist's work, commentators have noted its autobiographical nature and his concern with personal ambiguity and social issues. He often depicts a struggle between man and nature, sometimes with Darwinian implications. One work is actually entitled *Painting on a Darwinian Theme*, and was produced in the same year as this painting.

In this painting, the artist shows two hunters in an English countryside with the surreal sight of four lobsters on a rock beside them. They both seem somewhat confused. Behind them is a figure that is part human and part animal. The artist himself commented on this odd-looking individual, who seems to have been cloned from a man, a dog and a lobster. Could this therefore imply the results of a 'disruptive gene'? Perhaps it reflects our current concern with cloning and stem cell research into possible treatments.

A figure in the background seems to be peering into the abyss ... the fear of the unknown perhaps? Like much modern art, a superficial interpretation is not possible. But clearly the title implies a concern with modern genetic technology and its possible unexpected effects.

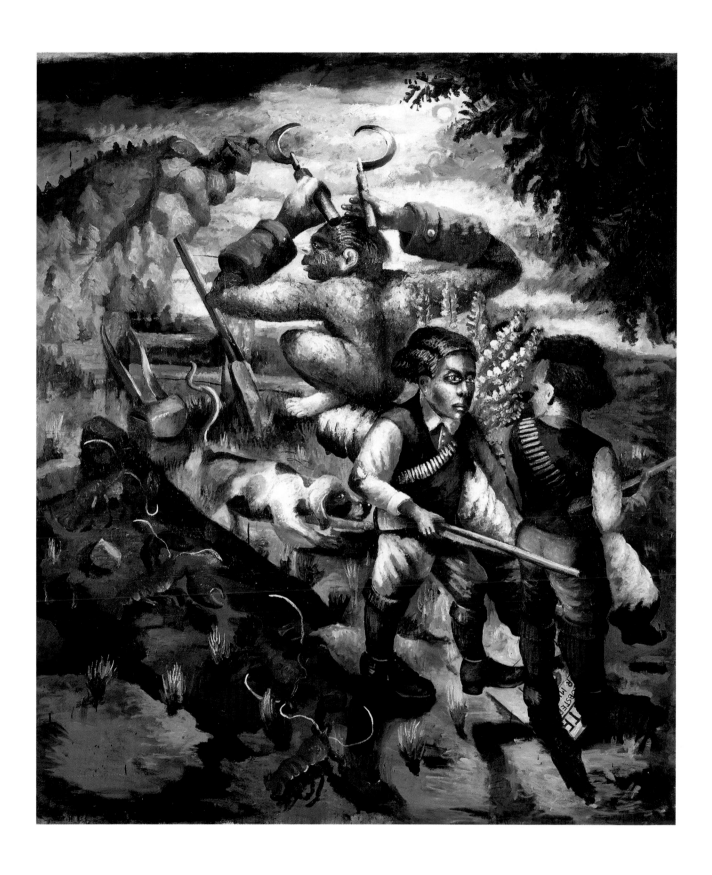

English Landscape with a Disruptive Gene (1987) by Steven Campbell. Oil on canvas, 250 cm × 236 cm. *Lisbon, Fundação Calouste Gulbenkian, Centro de Arte Moderna José de Azeredo Perdigão.*

63

Boy After a Liver Transplant (1989)

by Sir Roy Calne

Sir Roy Calne (b 1930) was, until retirement, Professor of Surgery at the University of Cambridge. He belongs to an exclusive group of surgeons who were also accomplished artists. He began painting at an early age, but a turning point came when, in 1988, he met the Scottish artist John Bellany, who was desperately ill with liver disease. Calne carried out a successful liver transplantation on the artist, who in return encouraged the surgeon in his artistic endeavours and advised him to loosen his style and use brighter colours. This advice had a dramatic effect on Calne's work, and he admitted 'I started to think of painting as a means of emotional expression as opposed to merely producing an attractive picture'.

This is only one of many of his paintings based on medical and surgical themes, but, as one critic has concluded, it arrests the attention with an urgency and conveys a message of compassion, tolerance and understanding that is difficult to escape. It was produced in the artist's studio from sketches made at Addenbrooke's Hospital, where Calne had carried out a liver transplant on the young man who had Wilson's disease. The artist has caught the relief that the subject experiences now that the procedure has been accomplished, yet at the same time a little of the apprehension toward the future.

Organ transplantation had been depicted in early paintings of the Saints Cosmas and Damian, associated with the legend of having amputated a diseased leg and then grafted onto the stump the leg of a Moor (Plate 11). There were also well-recorded later attempts at various transplantations, including a vogue for tooth transplantation. But all these were doomed to failure because of rejection.

The modern history of organ transplantation is associated with Alexis Carrel (1873–1944), whose technique of careful end-to-end suturing of blood vessels was essential. He pioneered several other important innovations and was awarded the Nobel Prize for Physiology and Medicine in 1912. Carrel had noticed that although autografts in animals could survive, allografts (homografts) failed. The answer lay in immunological tolerance, for which Sir Peter Medawar and his colleague Sir Frank Macfarlane Burnet were also awarded the Nobel Prize in 1960. Following numerous attempts to overcome rejection, Sir Roy Calne was one of the very first pioneers in successful organ transplantation, using immunosuppressant drugs for the suppression of graft rejection. Subsequently, many organs were successfully transplanted in humans, including the kidney, liver, pancreas, heart and various combinations of organs. In all this work, Sir Roy Calne has played a major part, not only at the bedside but also in the laboratory. He was elected a Fellow of the Royal Society (a rare honour for a surgeon) and knighted for his work.

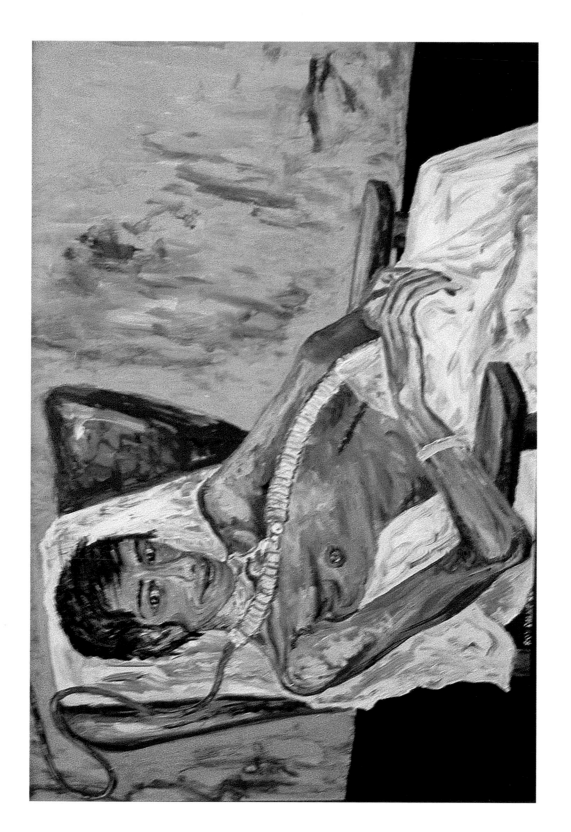

Boy After a Liver Transplant (1989) by Sir Roy Calne. Oil on canvas, 61 cm × 91 cm. Sir Roy Calne's private collection.

64

Cytogenetics: Studying the Chromosomes (1997)

by Susan Macfarlane

Susan Macfarlane was born in Sussex in 1938. After attending Winchester School of Art, her longing to travel took her to Sri Lanka and then to Hong Kong, where her painting really began. In 1964, she married and moved to France. While raising her family, she continued to paint, and during this period she was commissioned to design stained glass for the new Anglican Church in Cannes. She eventually returned to England in 1986 and became increasingly interested in observing people at work and their reactions to events. She then went on to produce two major exhibitions. The first exhibition, *A Picture of Health: Paintings and Drawings of Breast Cancer Care*, went on tour in 1995. It featured in moving detail the course of women faced with the diagnosis of breast cancer: the first consultation, breast aspiration and cytology, mammography, surgery, histological and other laboratory studies, radiotherapy, recovery, and finally the patient going home relieved and feeling good.

The second exhibition went on tour three years later in 1998 and was called *Living with Leukaemia: Paintings and Drawings of Childhood Leukaemia*. In this series, she traces all the stages from laboratory diagnosis (including chromosome studies, as in this work), admission to the paediatric oncology ward, lumbar puncture, bone marrow transplantation, radiotherapy, and eventually recovery and returning to school and later follow-up.

As Sir Roy Calne has pointed out in his Introduction to the catalogue, *Living with Leukaemia*, Susan Macfarlane's art humanizes diagnosis and treatment in a way that would be difficult to describe in the spoken or written word. Her works are full of humanity and optimism and will be appreciated by anyone, directly or indirectly, involved in these diseases.

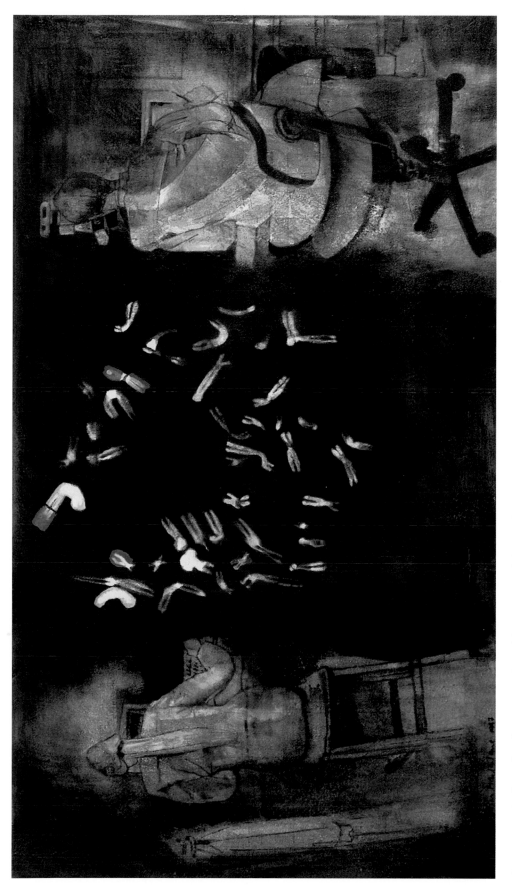

Cytogenetics: Studying the Chromosomes (1997) by Susan Macfarlane. Oil on canvas, 56 cm × 101 cm. *Buckinghamshire, A Picture of Health Ltd.* Reproduced by kind permission of Mr Euan and Mr Angus Mackay.

65

Three Oncologists (2002)

by Ken Currie

This commissioned work was painted by the present-day artist Ken Currie. Like much modern art, it is more challenging to the viewer than classical depictions of doctors. Such art can also reflect more of the artist's own philosophy and beliefs.

Currie was born in 1960, in North Shields and studied social science at Paisley College (1977–1978) before going on to Glasgow School of Art (1978–1983), where he was awarded various prizes and scholarships. From 1985, he became a full-time artist. His biographical details in the *Dictionary of Scottish Art and Architecture* (1994) tell us that he is a 'politically committed commentator, seeking involvement in the struggle for a more just society' and that he has a preoccupation with art '... as a social statement rather than as a vehicle for the expression of beauty'. As such, he is very much a product of our time. It is easy to accept these ideas on the basis of his works that deal with current industrial conditions. This large (196 cm × 244 cm) oil painting, however, appears to question the state of current oncology. The three specialists turn with some detachment to look at the viewer (the patient?) before disappearing into a curtained-off dark interior. Does the artist wish to imply that they are retreating into their own world of complex laboratory studies but are not entirely convinced or sure themselves as to what the results may mean for the patient? This may not be an infrequent concern among those who now find themselves having to rely on sophisticated and complicated laboratory studies for the treatment of their patients with serious life-threatening conditions, where always the hope is to find an effective treatment or cure.

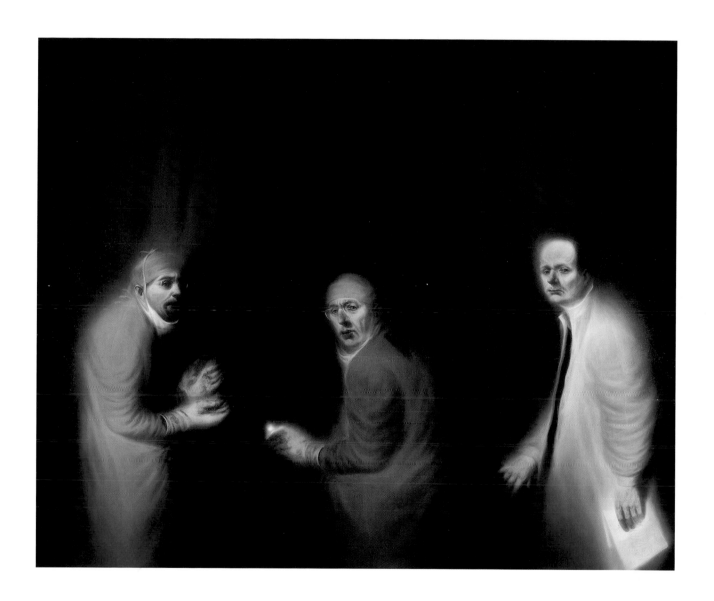

Three Oncologists (Professor R. J. Steele, Professor Sir Alfred Cuschieri and Professor Sir David P. Lane of the Department of Surgery and Molecular Oncology, Ninewells Hospital, Dundee) (2002) by Ken Currie. Oil on canvas, 195.6 cm × 243.8 cm. *Edinburgh, Scottish National Portrait Gallery.*
© Ken Currie.

66

Sleeping it Off (1996)

by Susan Macfarlane

This work by Susan Macfarlane is from her series *Living with Leukaemia: Paintings and Drawings of Childhood Leukaemia*, an exhibition that was first shown at the Barbican Centre, London in early 1998 (see also Plate 64). This series of works of art was initiated in 1995, by Dr Geoffrey Farrer-Brown, a pathologist who is now Chairman of the Trustees of *A Picture of Health*, a registered charity. The charity's aim is to promote art as a means of relieving the distress and hardship experienced by patients suffering from cancer and other serious diseases, and help to inform them, their families and carers about the illness and its treatment. Beautifully illustrated catalogues of its exhibitions on breast cancer, leukaemia and most recently on the heart have been produced.

In the *Leukaemia* series, an attempt is made to illustrate some of the situations that may be encountered by children suffering from the disease – and thereby allay some of the loneliness and helplessness felt in particular by parents. In this illustration, *Sleeping it Off*, the child sleeps after the lumbar puncture, and the nurse (but it could equally well be the mother), watches tenderly. In fact, nurses on the children's ward wear a special casual uniform to help children feel more at ease. The impressions of tenderness and concern remain, so like many earlier paintings on a somewhat similar theme such as that by Mrs Alexander F. Farmer over one hundred years ago (Plate 47).

Susan Macfarlane was a great artist who tragically died after an accident in August 2002. She has left behind a wonderful record of both the technology and the humanity of today's surgical and medical treatments.

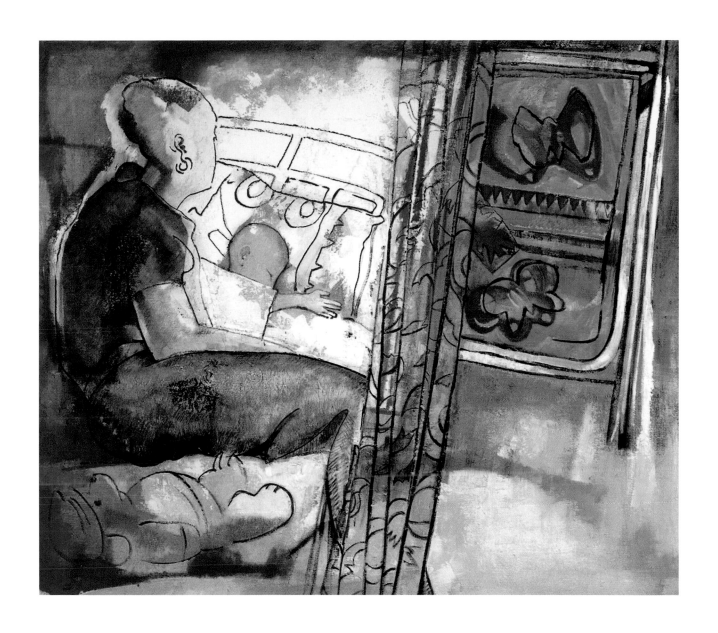

Sleeping it Off (1996) by Susan Macfarlane. Oil on canvas, 66.0 cm × 76.5 cm. *Buckinghamshire, A Picture of Health Ltd.*
Reproduced by kind permission of Mr Euan and Mr Angus Mackay.

A Selection of Various Surgical, Dental and Medical Treatments Depicted in Works of Art

(excluding those paintings described in the text)

TREATMENT	PAINTING Title (date)	Location	ARTIST
Auscultation	*René T. H. Laënnec* (? 1870/80s)	Bethesda, MD, National Library of Medicine	Théobald ('T') Chartran (1849–1907)
	Laënnec Listening to the Chest of a Patient (c 1910)	London, Private collection	Ernest Board (1877–1934)
Bandaging	*The Foot Operation* (late 1640s or c 1650)	London, Johnny van Haeften Gallery	Isaack Koedijck (1617/18–1668)
	The Good Samaritan [after Francesco Bassano] (c 1650–1656)	London, Courtauld Institute	David Teniers the Younger (1610–1690)
Bloodletting	*Egyptian tomb painting showing leeches applied to head of patient* (c 1567–1320 BC)	West Bank of Luxor (ancient Thebes), Egypt	Tomb of Userhat, Scribe of Eighteenth Dynasty
	The Surgeon-barber Jacob Fransz. Hercules and his Family (1669)	Amsterdam, Amsterdams Historisch Museum	Egbert van Heemskerck (c 1634–1704)
Chiropody	*The Corn Doctor* (nd)	Dublin, National Gallery	Adriaen Brouwer (c 1605–1638)
	The Pedicure (1873)	Paris, Musée d'Orsay	Edgar Degas (1834–1917)
	Chiropodist in the Bathroom (1908–1909)	Amsterdam, Stedelijk Museum	Kazimir Malevich (1878–1935)
Delousing	*Sight* (nd)	St Petersburg, The Hermitage	Adriaen van Ostade (1610–1684/85)
	Woman Combing a Child's Hair (1648)	Leiden, Stedelijk Museum	Quirijn van Brekelenkam (c 1620–1668)
	The Louse Hunt (c 1652–1653)	The Hague, Mauritshuis	Gerard ter Borch (1617–1681)
	The Family of the Stone Grinder (c 1653–1655)	Berlin, Gemäldegalerie	Gerard ter Borch (1617–1681)
	Mother Delousing her Child (nd)	Strasbourg, Museum	Michiel Sweerts (1624–1664)
	Interior with Mother and Child or *Maternal Duty* (c 1658–1660)	Amsterdam, Rijksmuseum	Pieter de Hooch (1629–c 1683)
	Mother and Child, With a Boy Descending a Stair (1668)	Bremen, H. Bischoff	Pieter de Hooch (1629–c 1683)
	St Elizabeth Nursing the Sick (c 1671–1674)	Madrid, Prado	Bartolomé Esteban Murillo (1617/18–1682)
	Domestic Grooming (c 1670–1675)	Munich, Alte Pinakothek	Bartolomé Esteban Murillo (1617/18–1682)
	Soldier Delousing Himself (1916)	Dresden, Kupferstichkabinett	Otto Dix (1891–1969)
Dentistry	*Tooth Mutilation* (c 400–1000)	Tepantitla, Mexico	Precolumbian mural, artist unknown
	The Haywain or *The Haycart* (1490–1500)	Madrid, Prado	Hieronymus Bosch (c 1450–1516)
	A Surgical Operation (1523) [line engraving]	London, Wellcome Institute	Lucas van Leyden (1494–1533)
	Christ Casting out the Money-Changers (c 1556) [left corner of painting, woman having tooth extracted]	Copenhagen, Royal Museum of Fine Arts	Pieter Brueghel The Elder (c 1525–1569)
	The Dentist (1628)	Paris, Louvre	Gerard van Honthorst (1590–1656)
	The Dentist (nd) [drawing, pen and wash]	Oxford, Ashmolean	Lambert Doomer (1622/23–1700)
	The Dentist (1630)	Brunswick, Herzog Anton Ulrich Museum	Jan Molenaer (1609/10–1668)
	Extracting Teeth (c 1630–1635)	Paris, Louvre	Gerrit Dou (1613–1675)
	The Dentist (c 1640)	Ledreborg, Denmark, Private collection	David Teniers The Younger (1610–1690)
	The Tooth Puller (1651)	The Hague, Mauritshuis	Jan Steen (c 1626–1679)
	Marketplace in an Italian Town with an Itinerant Toothpuller or *The Toothmaster* (1651)	Amsterdam, Rijksmuseum	Johannes Lingelbach (1622–1674)

TREATMENT	PAINTING Title (date)	Location	ARTIST
	The Itinerant Dentist (1654)	Amsterdam, Rijksmuseum	Jan Victors (1619/20–1676)
	The Dentist (1672)	Dresden, Gemäldegalerie	Gerrit Dou (1613–1675)
	The Dentist (c 1690)	Brighton, Royal Pavilion Art Gallery	Jacob Toorenvliet (1640–1719)
	The Four Times of the Day: Night (1738) [engraving]	London, Courtauld Institute	William Hogarth (1697–1764)
	The Tooth Puller (1764)	Paris, Louvre	Gian Domenico Tiepolo (1727–1804)
	Transplanting of Teeth (1787) [etching]	London, Wellcome	Thomas Rowlandson (1756–1827)
	The Dentist (nd)	Copenhagen, Medical History Museum	Francesco Maggiotto (1750–1805)
	Hunting for Teeth (c 1790s)	Aquatint from *Los Caprichos*	Francisco de Goya (1746–1828)
	The Tooth Ache or *Torment and Torture* (1823) [etching]	London, Wellcome	Thomas Rowlandson (1756–1827)
	A Coppersmith and a Tooth Doctor (1832)	Copenhagen, Private collection	Christian Andreas Schleisner (1810–1882)
	She Stands her Ground (1839)	Lithograph from *Grotesque Scenes* series	Honoré Daumier (1808–1879)
	The Village Smith as Dentist (1874)	Denmark, Private collection	Hans Ludwig Smidth (1839–1917)
	Dr Georges Viau in his Office Treating Annette Roussel (1914)	Paris, Musée d'Orsay	Édouard Vuillard (1868–1940)
Enema	*The Doctor's Visit II* (1670–1672)	Heemstede, The Netherlands, Private collection	Jan Steen (c 1626–1679)
Hospital care	*The Patients of San Matteo Hospital* (first quarter, 16th century)	Florence, San Matteo Hospital	Andrea del Sarto (c 1486/88–1530/31)
	View of the Old Sick Ward of St John's Hospital, Bruges (1778)	Bruges, Memlingmuseum	Jan Beerblock (1739–c 1806)
	The Convalescents (1861)	Paris, Musée d'Orsay	Marie-François-Firmin Girard, called Firmin-Girard (1838–1921)
	Dormitory of a Hospital (1889)	Winterthur, Switzerland, Oskar Reinhart Collection	Vincent van Gogh (1853–1890)
	Doctor Teaching on a Sick Child Before an Audience of Doctors and Students, New York Polyclinic School of Medicine (1891) [woodcut with added colour]	Bethesda, MD, National Library of Medicine	Irving R. Wiles (1861–1948)
	Hospital Ward (1920)	Stockholm, Moderna Museet	Hilding Linnqvist (1891–1984)
	Ancoats Hospital Outpatients' Hall (1952)	Manchester, Whitworth Art Gallery	L. S. Lowry (1887–1976)
	The History of Medicine in Mexico: The People's Demand for Better Health (1953) [fresco]	Mexico City, Hospital de la Raza	Diego Rivera (1886–1957)
	The State Hospital (1966)	Location not known	Edward Kienholz (b 1927)
	The Compassion of the Intensive Care Sister (1989)	Cambridge, Artist's collection	Sir Roy Calne (b 1930)
Mental disease (epilepsy, 'madness', 'hysteria', etc.)	*The Cure for Folly* (c 1480)	Madrid, Prado	Hieronymus Bosch (c 1450–1516)
	St Catherine Exorcising a Possessed Woman (15th century)	Denver, CO, Denver Art Museum	Girolamo de Benvenuto (1470–c 1524)
	The Extraction of the Stone of Madness (1556–1557)	Brussels, Bibliothèque Royale Albert 1er	Pieter Brueghel The Elder (c 1525–1569)
	A Quack Drawing Stones from the Head of a Patient (Dutch school, 17th century)	Rotterdam, Boymans-van Beuningen Museum	Attributed to Jan de Bray (1627–1697)
	The Quack (c 1656–1660)	Amsterdam, Rijksmuseum	Jan Steen (c 1626–1679)
	The Madhouse of Saragossa (1794)	Dallas, TX, Meadows Museum, Southern Methodist University	Francisco de Goya (1746–1828)
	Dr Pinel Unchaining the Mad (1876)	Paris, Charcot Library, Salpêtrière	Tony Robert-Fleury (1837–1911)
	Electric Shock Treatment (1908) [drawing]	Oslo, Munch Museum	Edvard Munch (1863–1944)
	Philippe Pinel Releasing the Inmates of Bicêtre (c 1840–1850)	Paris, National Academy of Medicine	Charles Müller (b 19th century)

136

TREATMENT	PAINTING Title (date)	Location	ARTIST
	Clinical Lesson at the Salpêtrière (1887)	Paris, Musée d'Histoire de le Médecine	Pierre-André Brouillet (1857–1914/20)
	Healing of a Lunatic Boy (1986)	Edinburgh, National Gallery of Modern Art	Stephen Conroy (b 1964)
	The Madhouse (1988)	London, Private collection	Sergei Chepik (b 1953)
Midwifery	*The First Morning (Albert and Charlotte Besnard with their Son, Robert)* (1881)	Los Angeles, CA, County Museum of Art	Albert Besnard (1849–1934)
	Romance, Self-Portrait (1920)	Edinburgh, Scottish National Portrait Gallery	Cecile Walton (1891–1956)
Military medicine	*Florence Nightingale at Scutari* (c 1856)	London, National Portrait Gallery	Jerry Barrett (1814–1906)
	The First Wounded, London Hospital 1914 (1915)	Dundee, McManus Galleries	Sir John Lavery (1856–1941)
	New Arrivals (c 1917–1920)	London, Imperial War Museum	Gilbert Spencer (1892–1979)
	The Interior of a Hospital Tent (1918)	London, Imperial War Museum	John Singer Sargent (1856–1925)
	An Advanced Dressing Station in France, 1918 (1918)	London, Imperial War Museum	Henry Tonks (1862–1937)
	Gassed and Wounded (1918)	London, Imperial War Museum	Eric Kennington (1888–1960)
	Bed Making (1932)	Burghclere, Hampshire, Sandham Memorial Chapel	Sir Stanley Spencer (1891–1959)
	Station Stop, Red Cross Ambulance (1942)	Washington, DC, National Museum of American Art, Smithsonian Institution	William H. Johnson (1901–1970)
Pharmacy	*Hippocrates Medicating a Patient* (13th century)	*London, The British Library. Harley, MS 3140, f39*	Illuminated manuscript
	Pharmacy (late 15th century)	Paris, Bibliothèque Nationale de France	Illustration from French translation of *De Proprietatibus Rerum* by Bartholomew Anglicus
	The Bitter Drink (1635)	Frankfurt am Main, Staatliche Institut	Adriaen Brouwer (c 1605–1638)
	Pharmacy (1638)	Location not known	Quirijn van Brekelenkam (c 1620–1668)
	The Doctor's Visit (c 1660)	The Hague, Mauritshuis	Jan Steen (c 1626–1679)
	A Man with a Vial of Medicine (c 1679–1680)	Amsterdam, Rijksmuseum	Arie de Vois (c 1632–1680)
	The Apothecary or *The Spice Shop* (1752)	Venice, Accademia	Pietro Longhi (1702–1785)
	Self-Portrait with Dr Arrieta (1820)	Minneapolis, MN, Institute of Arts	Francisco de Goya (1746–1828)
	Doubtful Hope (1875)	New York, Forbes Collection	Frank Holl (1845–1888)
	Drug Store (1927)	Boston, Museum of Fine Arts	Edward Hopper (1882–1967)
Physician and patient	*Physician's Surgery* (Athens, 480–470 BC) [aryballos or oil vessel]	Paris, Louvre	Painter of the Clinic (480–470 BC)
	St Humility Healing a Sick Nun (c 1316)	Berlin, Gemäldegalerie	Pietro Lorenzetti (fl 1305–1348)
	St Francis Healing the Leper (c 1630)	Milan, Pinacoteca di Brera	Giovanni Battista Crespi (called Il Cerano) (c 1575–1632)
	Quacksalver and Spectators (1648)	Amsterdam, Rijksmuseum	Adriaen van Ostade (1610–1684/85)
	The Quack (1652)	Rotterdam, Boymans-van Beuningen Museum	Gerrit Dou (1613–1675)
	The Charlatan (c 1652–1655)	Florence, Uffizi	Frans van Mieris (1635–1681)
	The Love-sick Girl (c 1660)	Munich, Alte Pinakothek	Jan Steen (c 1626–1679)
	Patient and Physician (1662)	Prague, National Gallery	Jan Steen (c 1626–1679)
	The Doctor's Visit (1663–1665)	Philadelphia, PA, Philadelphia Museum of Art	Jan Steen (c 1626–1679)
	Doctor's Visit (c 1665)	St. Petersburg, The Hermitage	Gabriel Metsu (1629–1667)
	A Doctor and a Sick Woman (c 1675–1680)	Location not known	Pieter de Hooch (1629–c 1683)
	Marriage à la Mode: The Visit to the Quack Doctor (1743)	London, National Gallery	William Hogarth (1697–1764)

TREATMENT	PAINTING Title (date)	Location	ARTIST
	The Doctor's Visit (c 1750–1755)	Amsterdam, Rijksmuseum	Elisabet Geertruda Wassenbergh (1729–1781)
	Death and the Doctor Leaving the Sickroom (1814–16) from *The English Dance of Death*	San Marino, CA, Henry E. Huntington Library and Art Gallery	Thomas Rowlandson (1756–1827)
	The Illness of Pierrot (1859–1860)	Kansas City, MO, Nelson-Atkins Museum of Art	Thomas Couture (1815–1879)
	The Sick Room (1864)	London, Coram Foundation	Emma Brownlow (fl 1852–1867)
	The Doctor (1891)	London, Tate Gallery	Sir Luke Fildes (1844–1927)
	Dr Paul Gachet (1891)	Paris, Musée d'Orsay	Norbert Goeneutte (1854–1894)
	Science and Charity (1897)	Barcelona, Museu Picasso	Pablo Picasso (1881–1973)
	Sentence of Death (1908)	Wolverhampton, Wolverhampton Art Gallery	John Collier (1850–1934)
	Physicians or *The Consultation* (Salon of 1911)	Douai, France, Museum Douai	Lucien-Hector Jonas (1880–1947)
	The Consultation (1922)	USA, Private collection	Édouard Vuillard (1868–1940)
	Dr. Mayer-Hermann (1926)	New York, Museum of Modern Art	Otto Dix (1891–1969)
	The Doctor (1950)	New York, Galerie St Etienne	Anna Mary Robertson Moses, called Grandma Moses (1860–1961)
Pulse-taking	*The Doctor's Visit* (1657)	Vienna, Kunsthistorisches Museum	Frans van Mieris (1635–1681)
	The Doctor's Visit (c 1660)	St Petersburg, The Hermitage	Jan Steen (c 1626–1679)
	The Doctor's Visit (c 1660–1662)	The Hague, Mauritshuis	Jan Steen (c 1626–1679)
	The Doctor's Visit (c 1663)	London, Victoria and Albert Museum	Jan Steen (c 1626–1679)
	The Sick Woman (c 1665)	Amsterdam, Rijksmuseum	Jan Steen (c 1626–1679)
	Doctor Taking a Young Woman's Pulse (c 1670–80)	USA, Private collection	Michiel van Musscher (1645–1705)
	Dr William Clysson Taking the Pulse of a Female Patient (1780)	Chicago, IL, Art Institute	Winthrop Chandler (1747–1790)
Purgation	*Man Vomiting* (early 5th century BC) [interior medallion, Greek cup]	Würzburg, Martin von Wagner Museum, Würzburg University	Brygos Painter (c 490–480 BC)
	La Source Purgative (nd)	Montpellier, Musée Fabre	Jan Miel (c 1599–1663)
	The Hydropaths: First Treatment (c 1880)	Bethesda, MD, National Library of Medicine	Charles-Émile Jacque (1813–1894)
Surgery	*The Surgeon* (c 1555)	Madrid, Prado	Jan Sanders van Hemessen (c 1500–1565/75)
	A Doctor Tending a Patient's Foot in his Surgery (17th century)	London, National Gallery	Imitator of David Teniers The Younger (1610–1690)
	The Operation (c 1630)	Geneva, Switzerland, Leopold Favre	Gerrit Dou (1613–1675)
	Shoulder Operation (1634)	Karlsruhe, Staatliche Kunsthalle	Cornelis Saftleven (1607–1681)
	The Witch Doctor (1638)	Valenciennes, France, Fine Arts Museum	David Ryckaert III (1612–1661)
	The Foot Operation (c 1640)	Amsterdam, Rijksmuseum	Pieter Quast (1606–1647)
	A Surgeon Applying Medicine to a Wound (c 1649)	Paris, Louvre	Gerrit Lundens (1622–c 1683)
	The Village Surgeon (c 1650–1659)	Oxford, Ashmolean	David Teniers The Younger (1610–1690)
	Barber-Surgeon at Work (1650–1670)	Mecklenburg, Mecklenburgisches Landesmuseum	Abraham Diepraam (?1622–?1670)
	The Good Samaritan (1737)	London, St Bartholomew's Hospital	William Hogarth (1697–1764)
	Avant l'Opération (1887)	Paris, Musée d'Orsay	Henri Gervex (1852–1929)
	An Operation by Dr Péan at the Hôpital International (1891)	Albi, France, Musée Toulouse-Lautrec	Henri de Toulouse-Lautrec (1864–1901)
	The Operation (1902)	Oslo, Munch Museet	Edvard Munch (1863–1944)
	The Surgeons (1912–1914)	Private collection	Édouard Vuillard (1868–1940)
	Homage to Mantegna and Sts Cosmas and Damian (1990)	Cambridge, Artist's collection	Sir Roy Calne (b 1930)
	A Liver Transplant (1990)	Cambridge, Artist's collection	Sir Roy Calne (b 1930)
Tracheotomy	*Le Tubage* (1904)	Paris, Musée de l'Assistance Publique	Georges-Alexandre Chicotot (fl 1880–1911)
Transfusion	*Child After a Liver Transplant* (1989)	Cambridge, Artist's collection	Sir Roy Calne (b 1930)

TREATMENT	PAINTING Title (date)	Location	ARTIST
Uroscopy and renal disease	The Consultation (1635)	Berlin, Museum Dahlem Gemäldegalerie	Gerard ter Borch (1617–1681)
	The Village Doctor (c 1650s)	Brussels, Musées Royaux des Beaux Artes	David Teniers The Younger (1610–1690)
	The Doctor's Visit (1653)	Vienna, Kunsthistorisches Museum	Gerrit Dou (1613–1675)
	The Anaemic Lady (c 1660)	Amsterdam, Rijksmuseum	Samuel van Hoogstraten (1626/27–1678)
	The Young Mother (c 1660)	Berlin, Museum Dahlem Gemäldegalerie	Gerrit Dou (1613–1675)
	Woman with Dropsy (1663)	Paris, Louvre	Gerrit Dou (1613–1675)
	The Physician in his Study (1665)	Berlin, Museum Dahlem Gemäldegalerie	Adriaen van Ostade (1610–1684/85)
	Visit to the Doctor (1669)	Germany, Private collection	Godfried Schalcken (1643–1706)
	The Medical Examination (after 1669)	The Hague, Mauritshuis	Godfried Schalcken (1643–1706)
Vaccination	Vaccination (1807)	London, Wellcome Institute	Louis-Léopold Boilly (1761–1845)
	The First Vaccination – Dr Jenner (1879)	Paris, Library of the National Academy of Medicine	Georges-Gaston-Théodore Melingue (1840–1914)
	La Vacuna (1931)	Detroit, Detroit Museum	Diego Rivera (1886–1957)
	Vaccination (1935) [wood engraving]	? Mexico City	Leopoldo Méndez (1902–1969)
Wound cleansing	The Wound Being Treated (c 1635)	Munich, Alte Pinakothek	Adriaen Brouwer (c 1605–1638)
	Wounded Man Being Treated in a Stable (c 1667)	Location unknown	Pieter de Hooch (1629–c 1683)